ADVANCED GUIDE
FOR PROFESSIONAL
HOMEOPATHS

A companion book to *Hahnemann Revisited* and
Achieving and Maintaining the Simillimum

DISCLAIMER

The information in this book is presented for informational purposes only. All therapies, treatments, or energetic interventions of any nature should be undertaken only under the direct guidance and care of a properly trained and legally qualified healthcare professional specializing in the services rendered. Nothing described in this book should be construed by any reader or any other person to be a diagnosis or treatment for any disease or condition. Neither the author nor the publisher can accept any responsibility for any ill effects resulting from the use or misuse of the information contained herein. Any uses or misuses of the information presented here for educational purposes are the responsibility of the reader. The names and other identifying characteristics of the persons included in this book have been changed.

CONTACTING THE AUTHOR

The author welcomes feedback from the readers,
mailed to the publisher's address below.

Full of Life Publishing
P.O. Box 31025
Santa Fe, NM 87594

ISBN 0-942501-15-2

Cover design: Marguerite Nastasi
Back cover photo: Yolanda De Schepper

ACKNOWLEDGEMENTS

The dedicated team that was at my side for *Achieving and Maintaining the Simillimum* has done it again! Teresa Kramer is my truly inspiring English teacher, who holds my hand lightly and steers me towards grammatically correct English. My accomplished editor Amy E. Lockwood, in her dual role of editor and homeopath, fine-tuned this work and asked me appropriate questions to clarify some issues regarding the content. The beauty of the work has to match the value of the information; Marguerite Nastasi is always up to that task. I am very grateful to these three individuals, who contribute to the homeopathic world in their own ways.

I want to thank my students for always pushing me to investigate new clinical problems and finding the solutions. And every busy man has a good wife beside him. I thank my wife Yolanda for her understanding and great support during all these years when I have had my nose glued to a computer screen.

TABLE OF CONTENTS

INTRODUCTION

I have finally resigned myself to the fact that I always will be writing, in spite of my previous assertions that "This is my last book." I am primarily driven by my enthusiasm to continually discover all the nuances of homeopathy, this magnificent science that enables me to treat patients in a more effective and more rapid fashion than ever before. For the good of mankind, I feel that I need to share these realizations with the rest of the world. Then you can decide whether there is any reason to be as enthusiastic as I am.

While I have already worked a great deal (more than 800 pages have been written) on my next book, *Beyond Jung: Delusions, Dreams, and Homeopathy*, I have found it necessary to temporarily postpone that colossal work and create a bridge, so to speak, between my previous works, *Hahnemann Revisited* and *Achieving and Maintaining the Simillimum*, and my proposed two-volume book, *Beyond Jung: Delusions, Dreams, and Homeopathy*.

As I constantly study Hahnemann and the Old Masters and follow clinical cases, I have experienced the need to correct, or rather fine-tune, some aspects of the homeopathic practice. None of these changes are my invention. All the credit goes to Hahnemann. I am continually astounded by the exactness of his words and his advice for the homeopathic practice. I hope to present these insights to the homeopathic world so that homeopathic practice may become more uniform worldwide. I also hope to assist the student, and yes, the practitioner, whether beginner or advanced, so that they can offer the patient what Hahnemann promised in the *Organon*:

> **A 157** The highest ideal is to restore health **rapidly, gently, permanently**; to remove and destroy the whole disease in the shortest, surest, **least harmful way**, according to clearly comprehensible principles (emphasis added).

Every one of Hahnemann's words still ring true! It is this fact that has motivated me to continue to look for "final" and "easy" principles to apply in the modern world. Notice that I have placed that word *final* in quotation marks. These principles will never be "final," but hopefully, this will be my "6th edition of the *Organon*," if I may be so bold as to make that comparison. I would like to stress that I never fail to take into account "*according to clearly comprehensible principles*," those principles that were so well outlined by Hahnemann.

I have endeavored to make this book a companion and extended guide to my previous books. This book, written for the practitioner and the student, will focus on four major issues that are frequent topics of controversy amongst homeopaths and have, therefore, a great impact on the way homeopathy is presently practiced. I not only intend for the reader to get involved and to investigate in an academic way, but hope to guarantee the clinician fast and optimal results.

The first issue will be to discuss *11 essential questions* the homeopath must ask after the patient's case has been taken following the principles set forth in *Hahnemann Revisited*. If those 11 questions can be answered correctly, the homeopath will not be led astray and therefore, the simillimum will be within reach. This information can be presented to any student or practitioner, and even someone who has not seen the patient in the clinic will be able to "see them." Many aspects of *Hahnemann Revisited* and *Achieving and Maintaining the Simillimum* are fine-tuned by answering these questions. They are like a final summary of observations that comprises all of the patient's facets, presenting the homeopath with the simillimum on a silver platter.

Part of the case taking process that is not only neglected in allopathic medicine, but is equally and surprisingly overlooked by homeopaths, is: asking about emotional traumas related to the pregnancy. These emotional traumas can explain the epidemic numbers of challenged children now united under disorder names such as Autism Spectrum Disorder (ASD), Attention Deficit Disorder (ADD), Attention Deficit and Hyperactivity Disorder (ADHD), Defiant Disorder Syndrome and Obsessive Compulsive Disorder (OCD). Many challenged children do not fall under any of these most prevalent classifications. Of course, allopathy is doing its best to come up with new disorders such as Selective Mutism ... but disease names such as this will never answer the two most important questions parents of challenged children ask: "What caused this disorder in my child?" and "What can you do for my child?"

While allopathy remains silent on the emotional traumas of pregnancy, it tries to address each "new" disorder with cumbersome therapeutic approaches that achieve limited success while demanding ever more resources, time, and money for all involved. Yet homeopathy has the answer to both questions. This book will help the homeopathic practitioner zoom in on the "first site of possible emotional trauma"—the uterus. The uterus, while generally seen as the promised and presumed safe haven or paradise for the unborn child, can be a site where plenty of dangers lie in wait.

Allopaths and many homeopaths have still not figured out that in addition to the miasmatic (hereditary) background, the uterus is the first place where the fetus can experience an emotional trauma. While allopaths focus on every physical aspect of the pregnancy, they still remain totally in the dark regarding emotional traumas to the pregnant mother that result in challenged children.

The second issue concerns miasmatic theory. As I read the *Organon* for the 105th time, I found that Hahnemann's discussion of miasms deserved a fresh look. I have learned to respect, to the letter, every word that Hahnemann set forth in his aphorisms. This, together with experience drawn from my practice, has guided me not only to a welcome simplification of the miasmatic theory, but also to a doctrine that I can use in the management of the patient. I previously alluded to this in *Achieving and Maintaining the Simillimum*; in this book, I will connect it to Hering's Set of Observations of Cure, the guide to true success in practice.

Miasmatic theory has not only been neglected in the homeopathic practice, but it is often denigrated by "eminent" homeopaths as nonsense and of no importance in the practice. Nothing could be further from the truth. This one aspect of homeopathy makes more and more sense in our ever more complicated world: it explains and predicts many disorders, behaviors, and diseases of humankind. The miasmatic theory is Hahnemann's most important gift to mankind, a concept far ahead of current allopathic genetic science. This book enables the reader to apply Hahnemann's miasmatic theory easily and correctly in the clinic.

The third issue, *potency selection* of the remedy, is the most contentious topic amongst homeopaths. No uniform opinion seems to exist, and harsh discussions often take place. Throughout the past 200 years, both camps, high- and low-potency prescribers, have been involved in heated discussions, both claiming that they have experienced success. There is no doubt that this is true in many cases, but is there a middle way? Is there a potency choice guided by common sense rather than passion? Is there a potency choice that can satisfy both camps because it is reasonable and effective? I wholeheartedly believe that there is. In this book, I propose a schedule that not only makes great sense, but guarantees greater success in practice. And all of this is based on Hahnemann's clear indications. Isn't this what a good homeopath wants? The best outcome for the patient and for homeopathy?

The final issue concerns Hering's Set of Observations of Cure. Was everything said by this eminent homeopath? Are there other observations that can help the homeopath select the simillimum and evaluate the direction of cure? Can allopathic terminology be used to "update" Hering's observations? Even

Traditional Chinese Medicine uses clearer and simpler terms regarding this Set of Observations.

While *Hahnemann Revisited* and *Achieving and Maintaining the Simillimum* have, among other excellent books written by dedicated authors, paved the way to the serious study of homeopathy, this latest book has fine-tuned several principles based on science and art, the latter being confirmed in clinical practice. These proposed changes are derived from using my newest methodology on myself, my beloved wife, my family, and on countless patients. Through my seminars, many of my students have already reaped the benefits of this newest information.

I believe that practitioners should read *Hahnemann Revisited* first, followed by *Achieving and Maintaining the Simillimum*, and finally, this book. This series of homeopathic clinical books will be culminated by my next book, *Beyond Jung: Dreams, Delusions, and Homeopathy*. That work will provide an extensive practical approach to understanding dreams and their homeopathic use, as well as a new materia medica of 100 polychrests discussed according to my core delusions method.

May you follow Hering's advice, "Don't reject anything without trying!" May success in practice be yours so that homeopathy can win the hearts of thousands of people every day!

KEY

A 157 *Organon* **Aphorism by Hahnemann**
This symbol represents the paragraph from Hahnemann's *Organon*, specifically the Aphorism number being referenced. Cooper Publishing in Blaine, Washington granted permission for quoting from the 6th edition of the *Organon of Medicine* translated by Jost Künzli, Alain Naudé, and Peter Pendleton. This edition was used primarily unless otherwise noted in the text.

Literature Citations
Much of the literature cited in this book is very old. For older books, such as those written by Hahnemann, von Boenninghausen, Kent, etc. the dates given in the citations are the reprint dates or editions. Please see references cited for more information on the original publication dates.

Quotations from Provings and the Repertory
Quotations from provings and from the repertory are italicized. I reference proving symptoms from Constantine Hering's *Guiding Symptoms of Our Materia Medica*, from Samuel Hahnemann's *Chronic Diseases: Their Peculiar Nature and Their Homeopathic Cure*, and from Timothy Field Allen's *Encyclopedia of Pure Materia Medica*.

PART 1: ADVANCED CASE TAKING

Forgotten Questions

In Chapters 7 and 9 of *Hahnemann Revisited*, I presented the great ground-rules for finding the simillimum set forth by Hahnemann. Each phase of homeopathy is a work of intense and judicious labor, which provides the homeopath with the nature of his patient according to the perfect prescription: the sum of Aphorisms 5 and 7. While Aphorism 7 talks about the "totality" of the patient's symptoms based on a value hierarchy appointed to the patient's expressions, one must not forget, as often happens, that in this same aphorism, Hahnemann also says:

> **A 7** ... it is evident that only the symptoms, together with **any possible miasm and additional circumstances**, must guide the choice of the appropriate, curative remedy (Aphorism 5) (emphasis added).

Indeed, without considering Aphorism 5, the homeopath runs the risk of dispensing a superficial prescription that might result in some improvements, but will never provide the desired long-lasting, deep-working actions of the simillimum. The miasmatic theory should be taken into account in order to relieve the burden of the genetic heritage acquired from the patient's ancestors (this theory is further explored in Chap. 12).

In addition to the miasmatic information, the patient's character, habits, social position, temperament, age, family relationships, sexual life, etc., must all be considered in order to separate the expressions of the true chronic miasmatic diseases (Aphorism 78) from those caused by allopathic intervention (Aphorism 74) or by lifestyle and environmental mistakes (Aphorism 77).

A deficiently taken case will only lead to a deficient follow-up appointment plagued by disappointments, loss of time and money, and worst of all, an acceleration of the patient's chronic natural disease. Homeopaths must heed H.C. Allen's words, "*A case well taken, is a case 9/10 solved!*"

The learning objectives in this book include *two new insights* that will greatly improve the likelihood of a successful practice. Firstly, the homeopath must pose *11 questions* **after** taking the patient's case. If these questions are answered correctly, then finding the simillimum is not far off. The homeopath has "the tiger by the tail," so to speak. Once these questions are successfully answered, different aspects of the patient will become clear, for example: the seat of the disease, the prognosis, the predominant miasmatic influence, the causalities, the different layers, the core delusion or main motivation behind the patient's behavior, the patient's temperament and constitution, and the source of energy leakage.

Some aspects in these questions are totally new and are discussed as a bridge to my next major work about dreams and delusions. Others were touched upon in my previous books. These *11 questions* guide the homeopathic practitioner to a correct or precise answer and give him confidence in his prescription, which brings success to the practice and happiness to the patient.

Secondly, a part of the case-taking process that has not only eluded the allopathic world thus far, but, to my consternation, has mostly eluded homeopaths—asking about the pregnancy. When the allopathic physician asks a patient about her pregnancies, it is implicitly understood that his main concern is the physical well-being of the mother and the unborn child. I do not deny the fact that the physician might be interested in major psychological events that would threaten his patient's welfare. In fact, the epidemic of "postpartum depression" has prompted several states to pass laws for physicians to watch out for this illness. But I am not alluding to these obvious mental and emotional states, which require early and urgent intervention.

What I am referring to is that allopathic physicians and most homeopaths do not ask the questions I pose in this book. Yet, the newborn's welfare depends not only on posing these questions, but upon the immediate intervention *during* the pregnancy, if possible. The most frequent question, "Why is my child suffering from this condition?" is only answered by the patient's honest introspection and the homeopath's diligent work. Correctly applied homeopathy is the only medical modality that can address this urgent issue of "challenged children," which has inflicted such a burden, not only on the innocent victims and their families, but also on society. Challenged children are the source of great grief, guilty feelings, and sentiments of helplessness among parents.

Homeopathy can successfully correct the situation right at the moment an "assault" is committed on the innocent fetus—right in the womb, a place meant to be a protective paradise. No need to wait until years later after the child has suffered physical and emotional problems created by what many consider as only passing occurrences and innocent moods.

The Art of Case Taking: 11 Questions to Solve Any Challenge

Extensive experience has shown me that many patients not only resent having to fill out lengthy health history forms, but are often offended by "intruding and private" questions that don't seem to have any bearing on their chief complaint (CC). Since a lengthy form results in an almost 100 percent failure and causes frustration and ill-feelings in the patient even before the first consultation, I suggest having the patient complete a shorter questionnaire in the office. The questionnaire can include the patient's contact information (address, phone number), family health history, and current medications.

I suggest starting the consultation with a casual conversation. While the patient completes the questionnaire, the homeopath can pay special attention to the patient's dominant function of consciousness (see Chap. 10). Remember that while a Feeling-Intuitive type of patient (*Phosphorus*) will be turned off by a "know-it-all" Theorizing-Thinking type of homeopath, the Thinking-type patient will be turned off by a homeopath who starts talking about spirituality when the patient's main focus is to receive a well thought-out explanation of his health problems. For a Thinking-type patient, the homeopath will direct the consultation from the physical complaints to the mental complaints and finalize with the emotional symptoms.

A Thinking-Sensation type of patient will most likely express his CC with a physical symptom, while a Feeling-Intuitive type will express his CC with an emotional symptom.

Since the homeopath will need to answer the following 11 questions after taking the case, he will have to ask the right questions during the consultation. Asking these questions will keep the homeopath on track and will enable him to share this information with others for either instruction or consultation.

---

11 Questions to the Simillimum

1. Where is the leakage of energy from the Vital Force (VF) or Qi?
2. What is the pathology and what system is affected?
3. Is my patient's ailment an acute or chronic disease? Or is it an acute exacerbation of a chronic miasmatic state?
4. What symptoms are common and therefore unimportant?
5. What symptoms are uncommon, peculiar, and rare (Aphorism 153)?
6. How many layers are present in the patient?
7. What are the "Never Well Since" (NWS) or "Ailments From" events?
8. What is the core delusion?
9. Who is the patient? What is his temperament, constitution, attitude, and dominant function of consciousness?
10. What is the patient's active miasmatic state?
11. In what miasmatic state of the selected remedy is the patient? Psoric? Sycotic? Syphilitic?

Chapter 2: Examining the Seat of Leakage and Recognizing an Acute Exacerbation of a Chronic Miasmatic State

Question 1: Where Is the Leakage of Energy from the Vital Force (Qi)?

In asking this question, you want to discover on what plane the patient expresses his symptoms? Questions 1 and 2 (What is the pathology and what system is affected?) help you address four important issues—prognosis, incurability versus curability, repression versus suppression, and nosology.

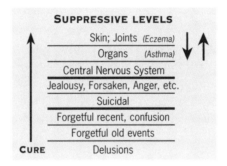

Determining the Prognosis

One question the homeopath (or any physician) will always hear is: "Can this be cured?" Even if the patient does not ask you this question directly, it will always be in his mind! Never answer that question over the phone until you have taken the patient's case.

Where allopathy has to confess (if they are honest) that they can only "control" disease ("take these medications for the rest of your life"), homeopaths do have the capability of curing diseases, even those cases called incurable by allopaths. This means that not only do symptoms disappear, but that the diseased terrain is eradicated.

Two noteworthy illnesses (among a whole array of others) are eczema and asthma. The interchange of these two illnesses, as seen in the clinic, is either caused by a changing strength of the Vital Force (VF) through various factors (emotional, environmental, etc.) or continued allopathic treatment that suppresses the superficially located illness on the skin. For example, the skin condition may move deeper into the lung. Traditional Chinese Medicine

(TCM) has understood this process for over 5,000 years. I have seen cases where eczema disappeared under the influence of cortisone and other suppressive therapies and was replaced with seizures, a deeper expression on the physical plane. The prognosis is much better if the disease is located on the skin rather than in the central nervous system or in an organ (e.g., the lung) or on the emotional plane where eczema might be replaced by depression or anxiety.

We must beware of giving false hope! Some practitioners promise a cure when the VF cannot deliver a positive response in a secondary curative reaction (Aphorism 64). It is here that knowledge of the "Second Prescription" is essential, as it will help you to recognize incurable cases. It can be difficult to predict incurability, however, and nowadays we can often cure cases on the borderline of incurability by using the LM potency of the 6th edition *Organon*.

Identifying Potentially Incurable Scenarios

• According to allopaths, reversion to normalcy is impossible when tissue, nerves, bones, muscles, and joints are destroyed (advanced structural damage). Examples include: blindness from optic nerve atrophy (in this case one still needs to treat the patient in his totality to save the other eye from being attacked by the syphilitic miasm); advanced cases of cirrhosis; tuberculosis; kidney diseases; cancer, etc.

Allopaths have declared many of these cases to be "incurable," but they were either cured by homeopathy or homeopathic intervention saved the patient from further organ destruction.

An example from my practice demonstrates this clearly. The patient was diagnosed with advanced cirrhosis of the liver with total Vena Porta obstruction and was put on the liver transplant list. When checked again by the Mayo Clinic after one year of homeopathic treatment, the obstruction was totally cleared. This created so much confusion that the technician reported to the physician that he had been sent the wrong patient as such regression had never been seen after allopathic intervention. Now, 10 years later, the patient is still alive and well and, of course, no longer on the transplant list. In all these cases, we must observe the reaction to the simillimum (assuming there is no obstacle to the cure—see *Hahnemann Revisited*, Chap. 14). So before we give a firm verdict to the patient regarding his condition, we need to wait and see their reaction to the test dose of the remedy.

• After administering the simillimum, the homeopathic aggravation of the patient continues for a long time while the natural disease progression adds many new symptoms to the clinical picture (see Chap. 12, Scenario #6 in *Achieving and Maintaining the Simillimum*). Only a few local symptoms can be improved, but amelioration of the general state or the well-being of the patient never occurs. This can indicate an incurable case. If the 5th and 6th edition potency selection and repetition is respected, this kind of homeopathic aggravation, in curable cases, should be zero or minimal.

• After administering a well-selected remedy, a short amelioration is followed by a long-term aggravation (see Chap. 12, Scenario #9 in *Achieving and Maintaining the Simillimum*). This is often the case in patients with extensive cancers. The administration of chemotherapy and radiation often turns these cases into incurable ones. I read in the newspaper about a cancer patient whose "treatment was very successful but he died from the effects of radiation." I would laugh if it was not so sad.

• After administering the simillimum, and in a case with no obstructions to the cure or miasmatic block, the patient shows a very short duration of amelioration in response to the simillimum (see Chap. 12, Scenario #3 in *Achieving and Maintaining the Simillimum*). We must make sure that a distant simile was not chosen. In that case, obviously, the complaint would be curable after selecting the simillimum.

• In spite of the simillimum, the symptoms follow the reverse path of Hering's Set of Observations, that is, deeper and more precious organs are being destroyed (see Chap. 12, Scenario #11 in *Achieving and Maintaining the Simillimum*).

• When exciting or maintaining causes persist, the potential for cure is limited. We think especially of the pseudo-chronic diseases of Aphorism 77 or "lifestyle and hygiene" conditions, or conditions due to lack of proper food and vitamins. We are not talking about malabsorption problems, which can be addressed very well by homeopathy. And of course, the primary maintaining cause is often a psychological situation from which the patient cannot escape. For example, a *Staphysagria* situation when a woman cannot leave a marriage for economic reasons or when a child suffers from domination and has no way out of the family. As Hering so eloquently said, "There is great indignation about things done by others and grieving about the consequences."

• Cases can become incurable because of the indiscriminate use of homeopathic remedies given in potencies that are too high and that are repeated too often instead of being judiciously repeated. Such cases are often more difficult to cure than those suppressed by allopathic medicines.

• When a vital organ has been removed, palliation is often the only thing we can promise, not a total cure. An example would be the removal of the spleen in Idiopathic Thrombocytic Purpura (ITP is a bleeding disorder due to a lack of platelets; cause "unknown"). What we can do in these cases is treat the syphilitic background so that no further destruction can occur in other systems.

• In the 10 percent of cases where an operation *is* necessary (obstructions, perforations, ruptures, and cephalo-pelvic disproportion in labor), a remedy is not indicated and will not resolve the problem. Rather, it would be more important to address the reason why the obstruction, for instance, occurred in the first place. An example would be the formation of scar tissue so often seen after abdominal surgeries. Years later, this formation of scar tissue can cause an obstruction.

I remember a case in my practice where a woman suffered from severe acute abdominal pain with all the characteristics of *Colocynthis*. When repeated doses of the remedy in water did not help, I sent her for further investigation. She needed very simple abdominal surgery. A single strand of scar tissue had strangled part of the colon; all the surgeon had to do was cut this strand. He never had an easier operation, but if such intervention had not been sought, it could have lead to necrosis of the bowel and even to death of the patient.

In all truly incurable cases, a palliative remedy can be chosen, *not* randomly, but still selected according to individualization, not of the patient as a whole, but at least of the symptoms concerned, including the pathology of the disease. The best way to find such a simillimum in these cases is by using the von Boenninghausen method.

Knowing on what plane the patient expresses his symptoms will also allow us to answer a second inevitable question asked by the patient, "And how long is my treatment going to take?" (although, again, the patient does not always ask their regular physician this question). Superficial skin and joint lesions should take the least time *if* they have not been suppressed for a long time (rare in the clinic) and *if* the homeopath understands the 5th edition *Organon* and the 6C split-dose method. Contrary to Aphorism 2, a fast, permanent, and *gentle* cure will not be possible when strong allopathic suppression (often with cortisone) has taken place. Only infrequent small doses and low potencies will be able to cure and exteriorize the suppressed illness.

Obviously, patients with frank psychotic expressions such as schizophrenia and many delusions will take more time to bring to a true cure. The homeopath must consult with the patient's psychiatrist to reduce (not stop) the allopathic medications from the moment the remedy "takes" or starts to work. The prognosis depends on the seat of the disease; the stage and nature of the disease; the diseases cause(s) and whether they can be removed; the extent of structural damage in organs; and, of course, the strength of the patient's VF. Therefore, a homeopathic physician should have adequate knowledge of pathology and general medicine.

A third use for answering Questions 1 and 2 is that they help us observe and evaluate our patient during subsequent visits (refer to Hering's Set of Observations). I warn you to act with common sense. If the patient's layer goes back many years and nothing but sadness and disaster fill their history, do not expect "happiness" to show up after the first or even subsequent prescriptions! A remedy is not a suppressive "happy" Prozac pill. What we can expect in response to the simillimum is:

> **A 253** In all diseases, especially in quickly arising (acute) ones, of all the signs that indicate that a small beginning of improvement or aggravation that is not visible to everybody, the psychic condition of the patient and his general demeanor are the most certain and revealing. The very beginning of improvement is indicated by a sense of greater ease, composure, mental freedom, higher spirits, and returning naturalness. The very beginning of aggravation, on the other hand, is indicated by the opposite — a more constrained, helpless, pitiable state with regard to his emotions, mind, general demeanor, attitude, posture, and actions, which can easily be seen and pointed out if one is attentive but cannot be described in words.

So this mental and emotional change comes *before* the chronic complaint disappears or the reappearance of old symptoms occurs. We must not forget that dreams, the messengers of the unconscious, often provide the first change that heralds the simillimum. Of course, Hahnemann says we can only expect this *if* the appropriately *small* dose (as small as possible) of the homeopathically indicated remedy has been given.

> **A 253** ... The signs of improvement in the emotions and mind can be expected immediately after the medicine has been taken only if the dose was *small enough* (i.e., as small as possible); an **unnecessarily** larger dose even of the most homeopathically appropriate remedy, apart from its other ill effects (par. 276), acts too violently and initially disturbs the mind and emotions too strongly and too long for the patient's improvement to be noticed *immediately* (emphasis added).

If mental and emotional symptoms were suppressed by the patient or by allopathic medications, the emotional symptoms will actually get worse after initially prescribing the homeopathic simillimum. This occurs because the patient gets "in touch" with his feelings. And if the emotions were not suppressed, because the patient had great awareness, what you can expect might be a lowering of the depth of grief with each judicious dose of the simillimum!

From experience, *Carcinosin* seems to be an exception to the above rule. Patients call it a "happy" remedy, because, often, the sleep improves immediately and anticipation anxiety disappears. More information about Hering's Observations will be discussed in Part 2 of this book. Since suppression is so common with our patients, it behooves us to see what Carl Jung had to say about this matter.

Jung: Repression and Suppression

I like what Jung has to say about suppression in his book *Collected Works of C.G. Jung, Volume 9: Archetypes and the Collective Unconscious:*

> The repression serves, as is well known, for the freeing from a painful complex from which one must escape by all means because its compelling and oppressing power is feared (1991, p. 63).

It is obvious that no cure is to be expected when suppression and repression, conscious or unconscious, of the complex takes place, relegating it to the shadow side or when suppressive allopathic medications achieve a similar repression. This repression is only a painful delay of the inevitable, as we have seen and will continue to see in the analysis of remedies. The return to the core delusion is guaranteed. Jung explains in *Archetypes and the Collective Unconscious* what has in fact occurred:

> The repression can lead to an apparent complete suppression, which corresponds to a strong self-control of the individual. Unfortunately, however, self-control has its limits ... Closer observation of people shows that calm is maintained at the critical moment [the moment they are confronted with the repressed memory], but certain results occur which fall into two categories.

> First, the suppressed [and also repressed] effect comes to the surface immediately afterwards [after the critical moment]; seldom directly, it is true, but ordinarily in the form of a displacement to another object or subject, i.e., a person is in his official relationships, polite, submissive, patient, and so on, and turns his whole anger loose upon his wife or his subordinates — his children! (Ibid, p. 63).

I have seen this many times in the practice. It is as if the patient is obliged to vent their anger and frustration on their loved ones.

This leads us to think of certain characters in homeopathy, "split personalities," who as children or adults can be "angels at work or school and devils at home!" It is also reflected in the rubric: *contemptuous, hard for subordinates and agreeable pleasant to superiors or people he has to fear* (see *Hard*). I would like to add to this rubric: to people he would like to impress or wants to be loved by. We see the remedies *Lycopodium*, *Platina*, *Lachesis*, and *Veratrum album*! All these remedies are graded a 1, and, of course, each remedy is "hard" for its own reason!

I would add *Silica* to this group because a person needing *Silica* can have a hard, stubborn attitude towards their family but be very nice and yielding towards everyone else once he leaves home. Hering said, "Child becomes obstinate, headstrong; when crossed has to restrain himself to keep from doing violence, and, yielding, faint-hearted, anxious mood." *Silica* does this because he lacks confidence and courage and does not want others to find out what is really present behind that self-assured mask.

What about the others? *Lycopodium*, with its great performance anxiety, is very similar to *Silica* (both have a "lack of spine or character" when unbalanced). A person needing *Lycopodium* fears confrontation with superiors, is easily overbearing to those he thinks he can dominate (like family), but friendly and cooperative with those at work. *Platina* is driven by her haughty delusions, thinking she has no equal in this world and therefore looks down on most people, unless there is that rare individual she can look up to. Consequently, she becomes socially isolated. *Veratrum album* is driven by *despair of social position*, so obviously they want to exert their power on those who are below them while they want to please those who are more powerful with the hope that flattery will eventually bring them to that desired position!

Jung also explains the second result of suppressing emotions (the first one being displacement according to Jung) in *Archetypes and the Collective Unconscious*:

> ... creates compensations elsewhere. For example, people who strive for excessive ethics, who try always to think, feel, and act altruistically and ideally [those we can refer to as being "unselfish"] avenge themselves, because of the impossibility of carrying out their ideals [or wishes linked to love, that ever-present desire in women especially] by subtle [and sometimes not so subtle!] maliciousness, which naturally does not come into their own consciousness as such, but which leads to misunderstandings and unhappy situations. Apparently, then, all of these [according to such people] are only "especially unfortunate [and unavoidable] circumstances," or they are the guilt and malice of other people, or they are tragic complications (Ibid, p. 63).

What rubrics and remedies reflect this situation? We can refer to the rubrics in the mind section of the repertory and to proving symptoms:

• *Reproaches others*

• *Hatred of persons who have offended him*

• *Delusions, pitied, he is, on account of his misfortune and he wept*

• *Ailments from being deceived*

• *Delusions, he is engaged in lawsuits*

• *Imagines to see obstacles everywhere, occasioned partly by contrary fate, partly by himself* (proving symptom of *Aurum*)

• *Malicious with anger* (*Natrum muriaticum, Lycopodium, China*)

• *Malicious, hurting other people's feelings* (*China, Tarentula*).

• The most outspokenly malicious remedies are *Anacardium, Arsenicum, Tuberculinum, Stramonium, Natrum muriaticum* (in its third or syphilitic stage), and *Aurum*, which goes to show that the brighter the light, the greater the shadow!

Question 2: What Is the Pathology and What System Is Affected?

We need to understand the assigned pathology and medical terminology. Patients (and their physicians) always ask the nosological name of the disease. In our times, we cannot say to the patient, "The name of the disease does not interest me and the name of the remedy is of no interest to you," as Hahnemann was famous for saying. Unfortunately, the patient considers the "name giving" the only criterion by which to judge the merit of his physician. While this is a very faulty criterion, the disease name will help the homeopath determine the patient's miasmatic state.

Furthermore, in practical matters such as death certificates, appearances before court, completing insurance papers, etc., a diagnosis of an *Argentum nitricum* colitis ulcerosa will not suffice, however accurate this might be in the homeopath's eyes. In these cases, the homeopath needs to understand the nature of illness in terms of disease diagnosis.

The common pathological signs of a disease are not very helpful in determining the simillimum, but they can help indirectly. The pathological signs and the allopathic name of the disease will help us determine the chronic and acute miasmatic state of the patient, which is the basis of our prescriptions in chronic diseases. For example, the syphilitic miasm is at work when you see: "destruction" (Parkinson's disease, advanced insulin dependent diabetes, Multiple Sclerosis, Alzheimer's disease, etc.); malformation of the bones (hydrocephaly, microcephaly, scoliosis, etc.); self-destruction (auto-immune diseases like Hashimoto's thyroiditis, rheumatoid arthritis, Crohn's disease, colitis ulcerosa, etc.); illnesses such as anorexia nervosa or ulceration from the onset of disease (ulceration not originally derived from chronic inflammation); and disease names preceded by the prefix "dys-" (dysphagia, dysplasia, etc.). On the other hand, overgrowth (tumors, cysts, warts, hemangiomas) and under-growth (hernia, prolapse, etc.) indicate sycosis. All functional diseases are psoric: due to a lack. The one exception is hypersensitivity (to foods, environment, etc.). For more information about miasms, see Chapter 15.

For any well-trained homeopath, it should be easy to determine the miasmatic expression of any allopathic disease name. Let's take the example of that illusive syndrome, Autism Spectrum Disorder (ASD). Expressions of ASD include:

- Avoiding eye contact

- Withdrawal from people

- Indifference to other people

- No facial expression

- Slow learners and monomania

- Aggressive behaviors: breaking, biting, etc.

- Mute (sometimes all their life)

- Echolalia or robot-like voice

- Freezing in position or rocking

- Change in routine is disturbing

- Rapid head growth

- Fragile X syndrome: 5 percent have a defective X chromosome

Although, when looked at separately, some of these expressions can be linked to another miasm, it is the totality of the patient's picture that leads to the accurate miasmatic diagnosis. For instance: "withdrawing" could be done out of timidity (which would be related to the psoric miasm). If it is one among several other syphilitic expressions as seen above in ASD, then we can safely assume that it is rather a syphilitic expression and not a psoric one. In this case, all the above mentioned expressions are linked to the syphilitic miasm!

Determining the miasmatic influence in the patient's case will keep you from making mistakes. In an example where we see sycosis in full bloom, it would be a mistake to propose a remedy like *Pulsatilla* or *Phosphorus*, both tubercular remedies. If one of these remedies *was* your choice, retake the case and have a closer look. In order to make a permanent, deep change in the pathology of the patient, the simillimum *must* match the predominant miasmatic state of the disease! In cases of severe rheumatism, we often find that the patient has symptoms matching *Rhus tox*, but this remedy is only graded a "1" as an anti-sycotic—it will not effect a permanent cure. We need to give strong anti-sycotic remedy such as *Medorrhinum, Thuja, Natrum sulphuricum, Sulphur*, etc. Another example is that of many asthma cases where *Arsenicum* seems to cover the attacks. But a true cure of almost any asthma case can only be obtained by a deep-acting, anti-sycotic remedy because asthma is mainly sycotic in nature.

Knowledge of pathology is also required for managing a case; for example, understanding the need for quarantine, for dietary changes, for rest, exercise, climate change, and prevention. A teacher with open tubercular lesions is not allowed in a classroom, nor is a high protein diet advised in kidney disease. A patient with Chronic Heart Failure is not allowed to go on steep hikes. When promoting prevention (better than cure!), we must also understand the nature of the diseases and their mode of transmission, as well as measures necessary for their prevention. How could we otherwise help our patients guard against these diseases?

The second part of this question refers to the affected *system* in the patient (expressed mainly in physical symptoms). Which system was affected first—respiratory, genitourinary, gastrointestinal, cardiovascular, or central nervous system? Why is this important? Each proven homeopathic remedy has an affinity for one or more systems—and each to a different degree. This information can be found in most materia medicas! If all the physical symptoms of the patient are located in the gastrointestinal system, then our simillimum, chosen on the totality, will take into consideration the Never Well Since event (NWS or "ailments from"), delusions, and mental/emotional symptoms, plus the main system being affected!

Let's consider an ASD case requiring *Natrum carbonicum*. This child will demonstrate over-sensitivity to milk and hungry sensations in the stomach at 5 a.m. and 11 a.m. (*Sulphur*). She has a weakness in the area of digestion and is thirsty during gastric upsets. It is here that the physical symptoms often point to the affected system and the simillimum. This is yet another tool you can use to check if the chosen remedy covers another aspect of the clinical case. The answers to these questions represent multiple check points—pieces of information that make our selection of the simillimum more dependable! If, at the end of our investigation, we have two close remedies, but one has the greater affinity for the patient's affected system, then our choice will be easy!

Here's another example. *Calcarea carbonica* and *Aurum* can be very close in their end stages (more advanced stages), as they both will exhibit a strong picture of depression. Let's presume the chief complaint of the patient is hypertension. We know that even the delusions of *Calcarea carbonica* can be close to *Aurum*. *Aurum* can have the delusion that *he is neglected* or *is not appreciated*, while *Calcarea carbonica laments that he is neglected*. All other things being equal, my choice for this patient with hypertension would be *Aurum* because it has a much greater affinity for the cardiovascular system than *Calcarea carbonica*, which acts mainly on the gastrointestinal system.

For more information regarding Questions 1 and 2, see *Achieving and Maintaining the Simillimum*, Chapter 12, pages 192-197 and *Hahnemann Revisited*, Chapter 13, page 251.

Question 3: Is My Patient's Ailment an Acute or Chronic Disease? Or Is It an Acute Exacerbation of a Chronic Miasmatic State?

The first part of this question appears fairly easy to answer. To recognize a true acute disease layer, make sure to follow Aphorism 73! If an acute intercurrent remedy is needed, be sure that you are not disrupting the chronic treatment unnecessarily (see Chap. 10 in *Achieving and Maintaining the Simillimum*). Note, that in general, any illness lasting more than six months is considered chronic. The appropriate potency and dosing most often chosen to begin the case is the 30C split dose as needed (PRN) for chronic cases—although high potencies *are* possible (see Chap. 14). Acute illnesses are often treated by using the split-dosing method with either a 200C or 1M potency.

The more difficult question is: How can the homeopath perceive that the patient's presenting condition is an acute exacerbation of a chronic miasmatic state, and that therefore a chronic anti-miasmatic remedy is needed in a lower potency—not a superficial acute remedy in high potency repeated often? Besides resolving the potency choice, answering this question correctly is important for another reason. In those acute cases that have suspended the old chronic disease (Aphorism 38), we do not take the miasmatic influence into account when choosing the simillimum. Rather, the homeopath chooses a superficial remedy

—

on the basis of location, sensation, modalities, and concomitant symptoms (von Boenninghausen method) so as not to interfere with the previous (postponed) chronic malady.

Two possible scenarios or ways exist that enable the homeopath to find out if she is dealing with an acute exacerbation of a chronic miasmatic state.

First Scenario

I have seen patients take *Nux vomica* as an acute over a long period of time each time they have lower back pain because it worked. In such a case, the homeopath and the patient have failed to realize that this is an acute exacerbation of a chronic miasmatic state, which crops up each time certain triggers ignite the condition. The homeopath should be alerted by the fact that this recurrent back pain is more often due to an emotional event rather than a physical one like lifting things. This may appear to be a recurrence of an "acute" event, but, looking at the patient's history, we find that it reoccurs over a lengthy period of time. The best way to resolve these situations is to apply the chronic miasmatic remedy; in this case, the patient would receive and 8-oz. Remdy Stock Bottle (RSB) of *Sepia* 30C, split dose. *Sepia* **is** the chronic complement to *Nux vomica*.

In order to avoid having the patient suppress his pain, the homeopath can give the acute *Nux vomica*, 200C or 1M, **even while repeating** the chronic remedy (*Sepia*, in 30C split dose, PRN). The chronic remedy needs to be given at a different time than the acute remedy. On administering the correct dose of the chronic remedy, there will be a rapid decrease of the acute events. Where, for example, the patient may have needed to take *Nux vomica* every two hours to get rid of his back pain, now, as we progress with the chronic *Sepia*, fewer doses of the acute remedy will be needed or, in the end, none at all.

Second Scenario

This patient will often present, at short intervals, *different* acute pictures (like weeds) that all belong to the *same root*. The attentive homeopath must recognize such a situation as an acute exacerbation of a chronic miasm, rather than falling into the trap of suppressing each acute event (see figure on p. 19) Let's take as an example with a patient who suffered three early miscarriages. The patient masturbates a lot, has an intermittent history of anemia, has involuntary twitching and cramping in the lower extremities, has green-yellow discharges (leucorrhea), and exhibits fits of jealousy. All these symptoms seem to come up at different times, suggesting different remedies. Some homeopaths try to intervene with different remedies suited to each acute event, as each picture rears its ugly head. However, when we look closely, all these expressions are linked to an active sycotic miasmatic state and *one single* chronic anti-sycotic remedy is needed to resolve all these manifestations!

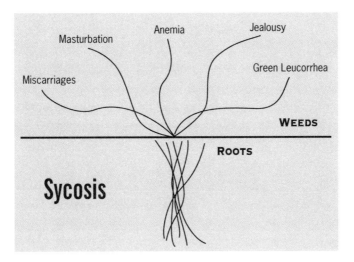

Homeopath be aware! Do not fall into this trap. Ask your patient if these "acute" events are recurrent and figure out which miasm they belong to. If they are all expressions of the same miasm, you recognize that you are dealing with an acute exacerbation of a chronic miasmatic state and that treatment must be aimed at the underlying chronic root.

What if the acute event appears to belong to a different miasm? A different layer has formed and a different chronic remedy must be found. If, despite good homeopathic detective work, the symptom picture changes at every visit, consider administering *Tuberculinum*, as this is a sign of ever-changing expressions of the tubercular miasm. For more information, see Chapter 10 in *Achieving and Maintaining the Simillimum*.

Question 4: What Symptoms Are Common and Therefore Unimportant?

Blunders in answering this question are easier than you might think. For instance, parents search the internet for information on their child's symptoms, mainly based on the nosological allopathic disease name. When the homeopath asks these parents, "What is your child's chief complaint?" they rattle off a list of symptoms they have researched on the Web. Unfortunately, this does not tell the homeopath anything special about the child in question. How is that child different from others saddled with the same disease name?

A good example is Autism Spectrum Disorder (ASD). The word "spectrum" should warn you that many symptoms are lumped into one "illness." Unfortunately, parents focus more on the listed symptoms than on the truly peculiar symptoms of their child—the symptoms we need to know about in order to find the child's remedy. Allopathy has the habit of setting up a list of criteria, followed by the comment, "If your child scores this many points, she suffers from this disease!" Parents think they have sufficient information when they list off the common symptoms or the allopathic name of the condition. If you tell them to forget the name of the illness and focus on their child's symptoms—how she presents the illness—they may think you are uninformed. (Examples of common ASD symptoms are slow learning, delayed communication, flapping of arms, over-sensitivity to noise, etc. See Chap. 2, p. 15.)

Some disease states keep the patient in an optimistic mood so that when questioned, he says, "I'm fine." Homeopaths recognize that a patient suffering from shock and uttering those words may need *Arnica*. For *Arnica*, saying, "I'm fine," is an Aphorism 153 symptom, but for other conditions it might be a *common* symptom. For example, a patient with tuberculosis who, after receiving a remedy, claims that he "is well." On further review, we find that his appetite is diminished, he has become weaker, his body weight has decreased, and on auscultation, his lung condition has deteriorated. The homeopath must conclude that the disease is worse, that the remedy was not the simillimum, and that the natural chronic disease has progressed, and so he must retake the case despite the patient's optimistic report. It is well-known that the patient with tuberculosis remains optimistic until the end: **optimism** is a **common symptom** of the disease! (See Chap. 9, p. 169, in *Hahnemann Revisited.*

—

Question 5: What Symptoms Are Uncommon, Peculiar, and Rare (Aphorism 153)?

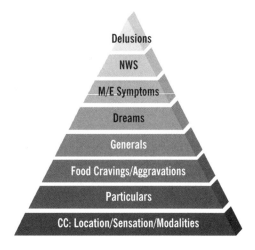

HIERARCHY OF SYMPTOMS

This question is fairly easy to answer. First, consider what is common behavior and then you know what is uncommon. I once asked 65 students, "Who among you would throw a chair through the window if you heard bad news?" Only one raised his hand. That reaction is unusual; the majority would obviously react differently. I was not surprised, however, that the person raising his hand would throw a chair through the window as a reaction to grief or bad news—he suffered from club foot, an expression of the syphilitic miasm!

Someone weeping at a funeral, for example, cannot be seen as being "*sympathetic*," "*oversensitive*," or "*weeping without a cause*." On the other hand, if someone cannot stop laughing at a funeral, we call this inappropriate and immoderate laughter, reflected in the rubrics: *laughs immoderately*, *laughing over serious matters*, and *laughing involuntarily*. We find that *Natrum muriaticum* is represented strongly in all these rubrics. For the rubric, *laughing about serious matters*, we see remedies such as *Natrum muriaticum*, *Aurum muriaticum natronatum*, and *Anacardium*. This shows that sadness often hides behind such contradictory behavior. These Aphorism 153 emotions are instinctive, involuntary reactions that upset the rational order of consciousness by their elementary outbursts. Aphorism 153 emotions are nothing but intrusions of an unconscious personality into consciousness. They appear suddenly, leaping up from an unconscious region, where they were disposed of long ago: such a "painful complex" needed to be banned to the unconscious as an act of survival. Primitive people used to call the appearance of such peculiar Aphorism 153 emotion (e.g., laughing at a funeral) a possession of that person by the devil or a spirit, and our language still expresses the same idea. People are almost completely unaware of the existence of the unconscious. The homeopath must make it his priority to go fishing in the unconscious to determine the patient's simillimum.

These uncommon symptoms take on a different value when determining the simillimum. Delusions, mental/emotional symptoms, plus general and particular symptoms, all can be "peculiar, rare, and strange," but they have a different value for the homeopath in determining the patient's simillimum (see *Hahnemann Revisited*, Chap. 9).

To help us determine the Aphorism 153 symptoms and rubrics in a child's case, for example, we must be familiar with normal childhood development. Of course, what are normally considered to be developmental milestones are not set in stone. With his knowledge of constitutions, the homeopath is not surprised that the stubborn *Calcarea carbonica* does not say a word until 16 months, but then starts talking suddenly in complete sentences at age two! Nor is the child who needs *Calcarea* in a hurry to walk or teethe!

The sexual milestones of the child are especially important and less known to physicians and parents alike. The pediatrician never spontaneously asks questions about the patient's sexual behavior. The mother is often embarrassed, ignorant, or hopes aberrant sexual behavior will go away, and thus does not mention it to the physician. You would be surprised how many mothers, homeopaths included, are in denial about unusual sexual aspects of their children!

It is of course necessary to understand what appropriate sexual behavior actually is. At age three, the Elektra and Oedipus complexes can be called normal, but if the object of love is still a family member in individuals past puberty, then we call it incest, a syphilitic characteristic and the source of many neuroses and regressive behaviors (*Hyoscyamus, Pulsatilla*).

This is what happens to a person needing *Hyoscyamus*: the libido can not be turned away from the mother or father figure, or whoever will fill that role, even you the homeopath. More than in any other remedy, overt sexual behavior is evident in the *Hyoscyamus* person. Of course, for *Hyoscyamus*, it is a "positive" tool to maintain his delusion, "I am going to be married." "I give myself fully to you," is the message. "I want to be on the most intimate terms with you, and no one should come between us." The patient needing *Hyoscyamus*, communicates with her "lover" in many ways that are not subtle. The following rubrics reflect the nature of a patient needing *Hyoscyamus*: *lies naked in bed and prattles; loves smutty talk; sings amorous and obscene songs; erotic mania accompanied by jealousy;*

onanism since childhood; has always been attracted to the opposite sex and prematurely busied himself with thoughts of marriage (delusion of a wedding); lascivious mania, uncovers body, especially sexual parts; goes about nearly naked, will not be covered; constantly throwing off bedcovers or clothes; entire loss of modesty; he lies in bed nude and walks in a fur during summer heat; desires to be naked and especially inclined to unseeming and immodest acts, gestures, and expressions; amativeness; nymphomania; and erotomania.

As the child grows up, it is very possible that such overt sexual behavior will disappear and be replaced with more cunning behavior because the patient knows better and has developed more successful ways of getting her way.

Children often touch their genitalia in the presence of others (Kent 698: *genitalia, handles*), touch the breast of their mother in front of others, drop their towel coming out of the shower in front of mom, or use sexual words (*lewd talk*). I wonder if a mother ever communicates this to her pediatrician. And even if she did, what would he recommend? A psychiatrist for the two-year-old child? Or anti-depressants? For the homeopath, differential diagnosis with *Medorrhinum, Pulsatilla, Platina, Origanum, Fluoric acid,* and other strong sycotic remedies is appropriate in dealing with such behavior. As long as the *Hyoscyamus* patient finds a sexual outlet, he is protected from total psychic breakdown or psychosis and paranoia, which is a deeper stage (core delusion, *he is going to be sold; delusion, he is being injured by his surrounding*). One of the possible outlets is that the child sleeps in the same bed as his mom, even at the age of 10 years and older. This often happens in cases of divorce when the father has left. If this cycle is broken, the child will show more violent behavior as his delusions, especially his core delusion, take over.

Treating these children before they reach puberty is imperative. Psychosexual maturation first begins in puberty. With physiological maturation, sex "invades the psyche" of the unprepared adolescent child. Psychological or rebellious troubles of adolescence are not pathological in normal children, but they will be accentuated in many homeopathic characters such as *Pulsatilla, Lachesis, Lilium tigrinum, Kali bromatum, Platina, Origanum,* and *Hyoscyamus.* The physiological maturation process coincides with the awakening of any pre-existing latent or dormant miasm. The mistuned Vital Force (VF) now has to fight against an onslaught of hereditary predispositions and is often overwhelmed by them.

Carl Jung mentions early signs of a child's sexual stimulation: making violent rotary movements with the forefinger on the temple, in the mouth or ear, as if she were boring a hole. Many of these children will practice onanism (the *Origanum* personality). In rare cases, as adults, they may fall into a schizophrenic state triggered by some unfortunate event. Jung describes such a case. A woman suffered from a depressive catatonic condition triggered by the death of her child, with whom she had identified through an overprotective love (Jung, 1991, pp. 139-141). Jung goes even further and relates biting nails (*Baryta carbonica*), finger sucking (*Pulsatilla*), and picking at things (*Hyoscyamus*) as symptoms of a repressed libido. We find these remedies in the rubrics: *gestures, grasping at something; gestures, picking at fingers; and gestures, playing with fingers.* For homeopaths, these three personalities all belong to the dependent remedies of Group 2 in the Periodic Table (lithium, carbon, nitrate, fluoride), or to needy carbon personalities like *Pulsatilla* (De Schepper, 2003, Chap. 5). A child or a schizophrenic adult may display less attractive symbols of welcome or declarations of love, for example, smearing the face and body with excrement (Jung, 1991, p. 185).

To find other uncommon symptoms, the beginner homeopath may try to notice whether the patient says anything that sounds uncommon and peculiar. It is always good to ask, "Is that how most people would react to this situation?" As Jung expressed it (see Chap. 8), the reaction to any situation is a response according to a fixed, predetermined hereditary pattern, *not elective*, but mandatory, which corresponds to our patient's predominant miasmatic state. An example might be various people's reactions to the same situation, for instance losing a spouse. The psoric person will look for consolation by phoning, talking, and emailing everyone he knows. The sycotic person might go to bars and drink himself into oblivion or might even resort to drugs. The syphilitic person becomes destructive (e.g., throwing furniture or tearing up pictures) or self-destructive (using alcohol and drugs that eventually make him lose his job, health, home, etc.).

Here's another tip to help you distinguish common versus uncommon symptoms: when you look at rubrics in general, the more peculiar symptoms are expressed in rubrics containing fewer remedies. Rubrics with 500 remedies (e.g., *weariness, prostration*, etc.) can hardly be called peculiar symptoms. But, the rubric—*delusion, he walks on his knees*—reflects the extreme bashfulness of *Baryta carbonica* and qualifies this as a peculiar symptom in a case.

A seasoned homeopath will not write down any common symptoms. Margaret Tyler says for example: "The more I practice, the less I write down." Her questioning would be geared towards the rare and peculiar, rather than the common. This is where the beginner homeopath can learn by watching a more experienced homeopath during live case taking. For more information, see *Hahnemann Revisited*, Chapter 9, page 169.

Question 6: How Many Layers Are Present in the Patient?

In addition to determining the patient's constitution, temperament, Never Well Since (NWS) event or etiology, the predominant miasmatic state, and the simillimum, yet another "diagnosis" must be made at the initial consultation. How many layers are present in this patient?

MULTIPLE LAYER DISEASE CURED

1 New stronger disease layer	**2** Older suspended disease layer	**3** Original suspended disease layer	**4** Patient constitution

Different layers are characterized by a totally different picture and casuality/trigger.

Before you decide on the number of layers, make sure you've thought through this question thoroughly. The true constitution (*Phosphorus, Sulphur, Calcarea carbonica*, etc.) of the patient is not a layer—at least not in my terms. It is rather the end phase of your treatment plan. **Different layers are characterized by a totally different symptom picture and trigger!** So, ask the question: "Does this or that symptom, that I would add to my simillimum, belong to a layer that has a different NWS than the one I am currently treating?" Various layers are usually formed by suppressive allopathic and homeopathic treatment and by denial of emotions existing in the shadow side. Layers are often detected by recording an accurate timeline in which each presenting symptom pattern, its trigger or causality, and its correlating therapeutic intervention are noted. We can also see the separation of layers because two successive layers indicate a different miasmatic influence. For instance, if the latest layer is syphilitic in expression, and the preceding one is psoric.

Above all, determine if all the diseases and expressions of the patient make up *one single story*! If the patient has a history of "forsaken," and the forsaken feeling was originally induced by the family (even in the intrauterine environment) and later by friends, lovers, and spouses, then this is considered one continual story of "forsaken," which has created one huge layer of abandonment. Only one remedy will be needed! I had an 80-year-old patient whose life-long feeling of isolation was linked to "abandonment" as a baby: her overworked *Sepia* mother simply put six bottles of milk in the crib for the infant to feed herself! The case was a long process of peeling this layer off with judiciously administered doses of one single remedy!

Don't forget that carbon people (*Graphites, Pulsatilla, Calcarea carbonica,* especially the latter) are stubborn, even about developing more than one layer. They often remain stuck in one layer and build this layer up for years on end! In practice, however, we are often confronted with cases representing many different layers in one patient. As always, the difficult questions are:

• How do I perceive the appearance of the next layer after resolving the preceding layer?

• When do I switch to the next remedy?

This will be even more difficult to determine when two complementary remedies are needed, since they have many peculiar symptoms in common. Remember, each layer needs a different remedy!

Complementary Remedies: The Difficulties of Separating Layers

Additional difficulty in recognizing various layers can be found when two complementary remedies are needed successively, such as *Sepia* and *Natrum muriaticum*. The homeopath may have difficulty differentiating a patient in a *Sepia* state, with her exhausted and confused brain, from the closely-related symptoms of the *Natrum muriaticum* state. "At what point is the *Sepia* patient sliding into *Natrum muriaticum* or vice versa?" This question must be asked in order to determine when a change of remedy (from *Sepia* to *Natrum muriaticum* or vice versa) is warranted.

It is here that the homeopath must pay close attention to any change in the patient's picture by comparing the core delusions and ailments of *Sepia* and *Natrum muriaticum*. Only then can the homeopath guide the patient through the difficult path that lies ahead.

In the following pages, we will differentiate between the third and final stage of these two remedies. Every remedy has symptoms that can be categorized as psoric, sycotic, or syphilitic. And over time, if a person is not treated or is inadequately treated, symptoms evolve from being psoric in nature to being sycotic, and finally, to being syphilitic (luetic). Luetic symptoms represent the third or final stage. The full-blown picture of *Natrum muriaticum*, for example, is not the naïve patient who is singing, dancing, and even shamelessly exposing her body, nor is it the excitable, dutiful, and dancing *Sepia*. These symptoms describe the initial stages of these remedy pictures.

Let's presume that an exhausted *Sepia* patient walks into your office. You will need to detect at what point a *Natrum muriaticum* state replaces the *Sepia* state.

DETERMINING WHEN ONE LAYER REMEDY REPLACES ANOTHER

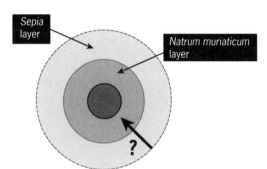

When you think the picture of *Natrum muriaticum* is coming up as the complementary remedy, but before prescribing it, you must make sure that the patient's altered symptoms remain permanent. Only when the picture is both altered **and** permanent (and after waiting a few more days) will you change the remedy to *Natrum muriaticum*!

So how do you determine the point at which *Sepia* slides into a *Natrum muriaticum* state? Let's begin by comparing the delusions, ailments from, and compensations of each remedy. Let's compare the delusions of *Sepia* in the third or syphilitic stage to those of *Natrum muriaticum* in the same stage.

DELUSIONS: SEPIA AND NATRUM MURIATICUM

• **She is poor (CD)**	• **Mother is dead (CD)**
• All alone in a graveyard	• Being doomed
• Three doctors come	• Will become insane
• Being laughed at	• Pitied on account of misfortune
• Being sick; will not work	• Being sick
• She is unfortunate	• Talking with dead people
	• Looks wretched, looking in mirror

Sepia has the following delusions:

- **She is poor** (core delusion)
- *All alone in a graveyard*
- *Three doctors come*
- *She is sick and for this reason will not work*
- *She is being laughed at*
- *She is unfortunate.*

These delusions reflect a sense of isolation while in a very ill condition. *Sepia* feels that she needs a lot of medical care (*three doctors come*), but fears she is not going to be taken seriously (*being laughed at*). These delusions show the burnt-out, exhausted *Sepia* state: someone who is unable to deal with work and relationships. Every small demand is too much: *delusion that she is sick and for this reason will not work*. Quite a contrast with the conscientious, dutiful, and industrious *Sepia* in the beginning, psoric stage!

Compare this to the delusions of *Natrum muriaticum*:

- **His mother is dead** (core delusion)
- *Being doomed*
- *She will become insane*
- *She is pitied on account of her misfortune and she wept*
- *Being sick*
- *She is talking with dead people*
- *Sees thieves in house*
- *She looks wretched when looking in the mirror.*

What does it all mean? *Natrum muriaticum* looks back at unfortunate events in her life: the split from her family (*mother is dead*, the core delusion), which also reflects the lack of *emotional nourishment* from the mother or *any* other nourishing source such as grandparents, spouse, child, boyfriend, mentor, guru, therapist, homeopath, etc.

The patient needing *Natrum muriaticum* has the persistent thought that she should be pitied because of all her heartbreaks (*she derives it from the way people look at her*, Hering). Often, the *Natrum muriaticum* patient will cry during a conversation with her psychotherapist or homeopath. Contrary to the rubric, *silent grief*; there is a longing to communicate with people she trusts or trusted or loved (*talking to dead people*), which also is reflected by the rubric, *homesickness*. *Natrum muriaticum* longs for the good old times, that is, they long for things as they used to be (for example, before the divorce, before the mother died, before her child died, etc.).

Increasing her sense of isolation, *Natrum muriaticum* is now convinced that she is sick and ugly (*delusion, wretched when looking in the mirror*) and vulnerable (*delusion, sees thieves in the house*; which, by the way, is not at all the same as *Arsenicum's* similar fear). With *Arsenicum*, this delusion is all about preserving his wealth and possessions for the future. With *Natrum muriaticum* it reflects a fear of bodily harm; that's why she has dreams of robbers! Again there is an extended meaning with *Natrum muriaticum* regarding this rubric. "Robbers" are also those people who intrude into her private life against her will.

The very first time a homeopath sees a *Natrum muriaticum* patient, he needs to gain her trust so that she will open up about private matters. If the homeopath asks private questions too early in the consult, *Natrum muriaticum* will retreat and clam up. *Silica* and *Kali carbonica* express a similar evasion (*aversion to being touched*). Such a person is literally horrified of being touched (too intimate). However, a good homeopath must "touch" this person on the emotional plane, and this part of the consultation takes extreme care and empathy.

The delusions of *Natrum muriaticum* do not include concepts related to work—only about *lost relationships*. Hering says, "*She tries to recollect past disagreeable occurrences for the purpose of thinking on them and indulging the grief which it causes.*" Here we see that long-lasting, unresolved, painful issues (oftentimes in women) that are related to love cause delusions (*no one loves me; no one cares about me*, etc.), fixed emotions, and fodder for dreams! Each time someone so much as alludes to this "high-feeling-toned complex" (in homeopathy this is referred to "ailments from" and reflects the essence of the CD; see also Chap. 6, "How to Find the Core Delusion in the Clinic") through a gesture or a word, she will react in a strong manner. *Natrum muriaticum* does not realize that she has become addicted to these negative feelings (*thoughts, sad, persistent*).

This is contrary to *Sepia* who struggles to get through the day, needs a daily nap (between 3 p.m. and 6 p.m.), and is indifferent to events around her and even her own feelings (*indifferent to everything, even pleasurable things*). It is difficult to differentiate at first because *Sepia* and *Natrum muriaticum* have common expressions at this stage of illness. *Sepia* and *Natrum muriaticum* are both

—

taciturn, offended at every word, and avoid company. *Sepia*, however, also avoids close family: *aversion to husband and children; aversion to one's occupation and family; and great indifference to one's family and to those she loves best*. *Natrum muriaticum* is usually in a precarious state as she has permanently lost these people (family, lover, husband, child, or pet) and now ceases to look for a new relationship and becomes a crusader for a worthy cause. She **still** wants to connect to "some" people, those who have suffered the same hardship. *Natrum muriaticum* derives energy from such a mission; it becomes her sole goal in life. She might even choose a profession as a psychotherapist or social worker because it allows her either to process her own grief or further suppress or postpone it. *Sepia* could care less (*indifferent to everything*). So *Sepia* is somewhat more challenged than *Natrum muriaticum*. The issues of *Natrum muriaticum* revolve around relationships; *Sepia* is all about **work and relationships**!

Let's see if this can be demonstrated through the provings of these two remedies, starting with the "Ailments from" or "Never Well Since" events.

NWS: SEPIA AND NATRUM MURIATICUM	
• Overexertion mind	• Anger/Silent grief
• Sexual excess/Pregnancies/Abortions	• Fright/Vexation
	• Deception/Betrayal
• Being laughed at	• Grief
• Anger/Business failure	• Disappointed love
• Emotional excitement	• Mortification

Sepia has NWS after *overexertion of the mind; too many abortions and pregnancies; from sexual excesses* (3); *from emotional excitement* (2); *from anger* (2); and *from business failure* (1). Ailments from business failure has an extended meaning for a patient needing *Sepia*. For *Sepia*, the NWS from "excessive demands from business" and even housework can also occur when she thinks that she has failed as a mother. Andrea Yaeger, infamous in the United States, drowned her five children in a bathtub while she was in the depths of postpartum depression. She had been plagued by delusions of being an unworthy mother months before she committed her heinous acts! We see clearly that the NWS events of *Sepia* point more to the demands put on her by husband, family, children, **and** business, or to physical exhaustion because of demands placed on her body (e.g., pregnancies). When *Sepia* suffers from *sexual excesses*, she has nothing in common with patients needing *Platina, Lachesis, Lycopodium, Medorrhinum*, or *Fluoric acid* who may have led a rather debauched lifestyle at one point because they sought an exaggerated sexual outlet in order to escape their core delusion. *Sepia* is not a highly-sexed character, but rather one who suffers from her sense of duty and possibly from marrying a very demanding husband in terms of sex.

Natrum muriaticum has bad effects *from anger; consequences from fright, vexation,* and *mortification; from anger with silent grief; from suppressed anger; from hearing bad news; from disappointment, deception,* and *betrayal* (3); *from grief* (3); *from disappointed love* (3); and *from mortification* (3). The ailments of *Natrum muriaticum* have everything to do with love or lost love—more precisely, with perceived or real deception and betrayal. Anger seems to be easily provoked by all this in *Natrum muriaticum*, but let's look at how these two characters compensate for their NWS. Perhaps there is another opportunity for the homeopath to differentiate between the two complementary remedies.

The Compensations of Natrum muriaticum and Sepia: Alike, Yet So Different

Sepia is quiet, introspective, and rarely speaks a word voluntarily; *she sits for hours occupied with her knitting.* There is an *inability for mental work*; it is even an exertion to think. If you ask anything from her at this point, she exhibits *passionate and irritable behavior since she is out of humor for all business.* There can be *violent outbursts of anger at that moment, especially when she is contradicted. She felt all day like she did not care what happened,* and there is *great indifference to everything.* Here is another difference with *Natrum muriaticum*: in *Sepia* there is *frequent weeping which she can scarcely suppress, every few minutes inclined to cry, without knowing the cause. Sepia* cries more than anyone in our materia medica, even more than *Pulsatilla.*

Leave *Sepia* alone and she is OK! *Sepia* wants a **vacation**, whereas *Natrum muriaticum* wants a **vocation**! *Sepia* won't get involved in any project or good cause as does *Natrum muriaticum*—at this point, *Sepia* just doesn't care!

Natrum muriaticum loves classical music as it resonates with her, Sepia has aggravation from music (except in the first stage where dancing is a way for *Sepia* to deal with the feeling of stagnation). *Sepia cries when telling her symptoms. Natrum muriaticum* suppresses her symptoms and does not cry when telling her symptoms unless she believes she is pitied. *Natrum muriaticum* is much more passionate about trifles and has a hateful and vindictive nature. *Sepia,* on the other hand, has indifference to everything. *Natrum muriaticum* has palpitations and headaches in the morning upon awaking (compare to *Lachesis*).

One can see how much attention is necessary before the homeopath can decide that a *Sepia* situation has turned into a *Natrum muriaticum* situation. The great

—

giveaway is the following. When the patient is in a *Sepia* state, you know there are professional **and** relationship problems! When you think *Natrum muriaticum* is showing up in the patient's picture, and its symptoms remain persistent, ask how the patient is doing at work. She might answer: "At work everything is fine now!" Maybe she got another job or a different boss, etc. But her personal relationships with husband, friend, parent, child, etc. are still difficult. At that point you know that there is a great possibility you need to switch the remedy to *Natrum muriaticum*.

The Appropriate Acute Remedy May Show Us the Way

Besides paying attention to these differences in delusions, NWS events, and compensations, how can we further distinguish these different layers? One possible way is by detecting the need to give the complementary remedy: that is, an acute situation shows up, pointing to a simillimum that is the **acute** remedy of the next, complementary chronic one. For example, a patient is taking *Sepia*, but now gets headaches from being in the sun. Repeated doses of *Sepia* do not help, nor does *Nux vomica*, the acute of *Sepia*, provide relief. But *Bryonia* (the acute of *Natrum muriaticum*) resolves the headache in minutes! Or pain in the right ovary responds nicely to a dose of *Apis* (another acute of *Natrum muriaticum*) or edema around the eyes is improved by a dose of *Apis*. We begin to suspect that *Natrum muriaticum* is either already needed or that we are now very close to the layer needing *Natrum muriaticum*! Perhaps the patient complains about a recurrence of fever blisters (herpes simplex I), water retention, and weight gain, all indications of *Natrum muriaticum*. And now she becomes more verbal in expressing her dislike of those *who have offended her in the past*. When these symptoms remain permanent—lasting at least a week rather than one day—*Natrum muriaticum* must be seriously considered for this patient.

On the contrary, when sliding from a *Natrum muriaticum* into a *Sepia* state, the first symptoms indicating *Sepia* might be acute lower back pain and fainting, as well as behaving very irritably, even towards those she loves the most—her children and husband.

Remember that the symptoms must remain in a permanent state in order to indicate the next chronic remedy layer, but just the appearance of certain symptoms tells you that the patient is getting closer to the next remedy, so that repetition of the previous chronic remedy should be undertaken with care. For more information, see *Hahnemann Revisited*, Chapter 10, page 207 and *Achieving and Maintaining the Simillimum*, Chapter 13, page 201.

—

Must the Patient Suffer While the Remedy Works?

This brings up another issue regarding case management. One of my students asked the following question and partly answered it herself. The student needed clarification after reading about the primary action and the curative counter-action (Aphorisms 63-64).

Student's questions: "Is it true that sensitive patients will always experience some sort of curative counteraction that is uncomfortable? Say, for instance, that a client on anti-depressants and narcotic pain medication needs *Ignatia*. You give a low potency and a small dose (e.g., a 6C potency using the split-dose method and only one succussion to the bottle; or have the patient smell the remedy—olfaction method). If the patient has a strong enough Vital Force (VF), she may become weepy and somewhat irrational, which is seen by the patient as threatening to her emotional balance. Of course, what the practitioner sees is the similar aggravation of the remedy—leading to the curative counteraction. Is the remedy strong enough to produce an action deeper than the allopathic drugs?

"For any patient, especially the sensitive patient, giving *Ignatia* may integrate suppressed grief and indignation from the unconsciousness to the consciousness, which is obviously painful and counteracts the numbing effects of the allopathic medications. So, do we lower the potency, limit the exposure to the remedy, succuss only once, or what?

"In Aphorism 69," my student continued, "Hahnemann states that *the antipathic remedy masks the opposite natural disease symptoms only superficially*. If the client never wanted to feel the 'pain' of her grief, then any curative counteraction will be felt as something threatening, because it is not 'superficial' but curative.

"Is it possible to completely extinguish the discomfort of the remedy's action by lowering the potency even more? Is there a point where 'no pain, no gain' is true to some extent? In a way, it reminds me of an 'intervention' (in other words, the 'pain' may be uncomfortable but it can lead to a healthier, happier life)."

Dr. Luc's answer: "Hahnemann is quite correct in these aphorisms: it is very difficult, perhaps impossible, to make the dose so small that no **psychological discomfort** occurs. This is NOT related to a similar aggravation, but rather to the awakening of suppressed emotions. Of course, it hurts when such feelings resurface, but the continued judicious intake of the remedy will help the patient move forward! The antipathic (allopathic) unnatural therapy makes the patient numb or in other words, stagnant, as the drugs kill any emotional freedom left in him!

—

"We find this even in physical problems. Take the case of a *Helleborus* stroke: as the patient 'comes to life' again, his numbness will become painful tingling, heralding a return to life of the physical body. You can compare this to the emotional awakening of the body. Of course, we don't want to do what Kent did, administering *Helleborus* 10M to a child who then screamed with pain while coming out of unconsciousness far too fast (see Kent, J.T., *Lectures on Materia Medica*, p. 517). Hahnemann's 5th edition split-dose method will minimize discomfort, but discomfort there will be! Do we adjust the dose and/or potency? Only if the suppressed symptoms are too severe!

"We see this situation often in the case of hemiplegia or stroke. Under the influence of the simillimum, the initial paralysis will go from great numbness to strong, even painful tingling. While we are rejoicing in this evolution, because it is proceeding toward a cure, the patient may suffer more than necessary if the homeopath is not able to adjust the dose/frequency of administration of the simillimum. Luckily, we have the 5th and 6th editions of the *Organon* which offers methods that can lessen this suffering!

"A special incidence can surface during the treatment of a suppressed psychological state, for example, a case of long-term suppression, possibly a situation requiring *Staphysagria*. Judicious doses of *Staphysagria*, even using the 5th edition split-dose method, might bring up well-hidden feelings of anger and sadness very rapidly, and the patient may claim to be "very sensitive" to this remedy. It is here that additional adjustments of the *dose*, which can never be too small if it is indeed the simillimum (see *Chronic Diseases*, Hahnemann, Volume I, p. 120; see also Chap. 14) and repetition are necessary. I have also noticed that these patients become more sensitive to anything in the environment: smells, toxic substances, etc. It is as if the reawakening of emotions in a person who has been numb for so many years leads to a general reawakening of the senses that now have difficulty coping with the challenge. You can compare this to someone who has been sequestered in the darkness for years and must now face daylight. What is tolerable to someone else is torture to them! This reawakening of the senses is following the direction of cure according to Hering. And we also see progression from numbness/paralysis, which is syphilitic in nature, to hypersensitivity, a psoric condition. This direction of cure from syphilitic to psoric is yet another indication of healing. Besides making sure that the dose remains as small as possible (perhaps even reducing it to drops) and that the interval between doses is well chosen, the homeopath should keep the number of succussions high and possibly even increase the potency of the remedy (from 6C to 30C) as the patient's VF shows improved reactivity and now needs more support (see Chap. 14)."

—

Student's second question: The previous discussion prompted another excellent question from a student. "How do you differentiate between a similar aggravation and 'psychological discomfort'?"

Logically, a similar aggravation would come from the primary action of the remedy (the remedy is too strong). Psychological discomfort is a secondary action, presumably caused by the VF.

PRIMARY AND SEONDARY ACTIONS OF A REMEDY

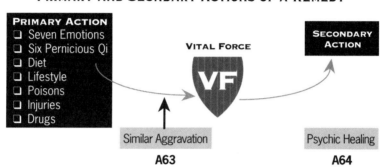

The student went on to say: "When talking to patients and trying to interpret the action of the remedy, I can't seem to distinguish the difference through the symptoms they express, so I am unsure how to manage the case. It becomes even harder to distinguish when the patient's symptoms are past symptoms **and** the symptoms expressed are also symptoms of the remedy. I was working yesterday with a patient who had upped the number of succussions of her chronic remedy for menopausal symptoms (*Lachesis*) a few days before. Since then she had been feeling unloved, unwanted, not appreciated, and unsupported. With fewer succussions she didn't have those feelings, but it also didn't seem that anything was happening with the remedy at that potency. She acknowledges having had those feelings in the past. Do we continue with the remedy at the higher level of succussion, according to the 'no pain, no gain' philosophy, or should we lower the dose, a second option, because the symptoms may be a similar aggravation caused by the remedy?"

Dr. Luc's answer: "We are talking here about the correct interpretation of Hering's Set of Observations. There are two possibilities. The emotional symptoms may still belong to the layer you are treating (return of old symptoms). In this case you must, in fact, continue with the previous number of succussions and the amount of the dose. Explain carefully to the patient what is happening. Remember that a simple sketch may aid understanding. You cannot let the patient remain stagnant in a 'bad place.' You must move the case forward."

PATIENT'S HEALING PROCESS

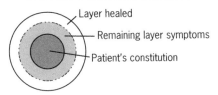

Layer healed
Remaining layer symptoms
Patient's constitution

Psychological pain originates from the resolution of suppressed and repressed emotions and is indeed a result of the secondary action of the remedy (Aphorism 64). The similar aggravation is indeed a consequence of the primary action of the remedy (Aphorism 63)!

This question is really an issue when we are talking about a "psychological" pain and not a "physical" pain. Healing physically affects people differently: the sycotic person, for example, always heals slowly on the physical plane. On the "physical plane," I would say, "no pain, MORE gain." Just think about people who wreak havoc on their bodies by over-exercising when lifting weights, etc. We do not want to imitate practitioners using 4th edition methods—those who **want** to see a similar aggravation. In the case of old physical symptoms, therefore, the return of old symptoms must be held to a minimum of intensity and duration through manipulation of the dose and potency (easily done with the 5th edition split-dose method).

The question remains: What if the chief complaint (CC) is a psychological problem, for example, jealousy?

Since *Lachesis* was the remedy given to the student's patient, what if the person reacts with even more jealousy after a dose? How do we distinguish between a psychological disturbance (or reappearance of old feelings) and a similar aggravation, since jealousy is obviously a proving symptom of *Lachesis*? This is mainly a question of the *time of onset of the "aggravation." A similar aggravation will occur within a day if not sooner; a return* of old symptoms takes longer to appear. If we take the example of jealousy: a *return of old symptoms* will often take the same form as it did in old instances of jealousy. When you are dealing with similar aggravation, however, other instances of jealousy and especially other emotional expressions belonging to the proving symptoms (*anticipation anxiety, restlessness, melancholy, and easily offended*) might accompany the jealous behavior.Let's say that before this patient took her dose, she felt "in balance" emotionally, having relegated her "sensitive characteristics" to her shadow side. Now, under the influence of the simillimum, this "false and frail balance" is broken, since it was only a well-formed compensation.

In addition, there is another issue, which requires a totally different homeopathic approach. I find that my students experience considerable difficulty when it comes to separating layers in their patients' cases. We know that, according to Hering's Set of Observations, when old symptoms return, the remedy should not be changed but instead continued in order to bring about a cure. However, this is not the same thing as symptoms returning from the next untreated layer. As mentioned above, this **is** a different layer, with a different NWS and a different set of symptoms from the one my student had been treating recently (the *Lachesis* layer). The original CC of my student's patient was extreme jealousy around the time of her menopause. The totality of the symptoms of this patient pointed to *Lachesis*. After a period of treatment with *Lachesis*, which successfully eliminated these symptoms in the patient, she now complained of feeling that she could not succeed at anything; everything would fail. She felt quite tearful and trapped in her situation. These were old symptoms that she had felt for part of her life.

Because "there is a return of old symptoms," we might believe that we must continue with *Lachesis*. However, the delusions or fixed ideas that this patient now expresses (delusions: *she cannot succeed, she does everything wrong; she will fail; she does nothing right; is unfit for this world; she is worthless*; and *fear of failure*) all point to *Aurum*! These are new symptoms, and it would be prudent at this point to look in her past medical history to see if there were other ailments belonging to *Aurum* (*grief, loss of money, hearing bad news, disappointed love*). When my student reexamined this case on my advice, she found other characteristics of *Aurum*: extreme guilt about "failing" as a mother and spouse (although the patient was not in fact at fault), which easily gives birth to the delusion, *neglected her duty*. And indeed, plenty of examples of the NWS of *Aurum* were also present: *disappointed love, grief, fright, being scorned*, and *violence*. This should make the homeopath realize that these old "returning" symptoms **do** in fact belong to the next layer, and a different remedy **is** needed!

DISCOVERING DIFFERENT LAYERS

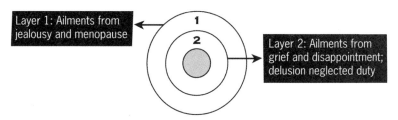

Here is what the patient in question reported after the first dose of *Aurum*:

> I really like my *Aurum*. I had my best bike ride in about a year after the dose and played my best-ever game of racquet ball today. My husband and I were goofing around and laughing so hard, I felt like someone gave me a silly pill. Here is the best part: my libido seems to have returned after being pretty much absent for some time! I also have been feeling very upbeat overall.

This is a clear reaction to the simillimum. This stresses again that we really must **treat the active disease layer** of the patient! What would have happened if we had continued with *Lachesis*? The formation of a complex disease (Aphorism 40), a more difficult condition to treat.

Chapter 5: The Etiology

Question 7: What Are the NWS or "Ailments From" Events?

NWS and the Formation of Delusions

Identifying the causality, in homeopathic terms, is the second most valuable symptom in your search for the simillimum. The core and secondary delusions are the most valuable symptoms. What triggered the onset of symptoms? Make sure that you link this trigger to the first layer you will treat!

Often the trigger can be expressed by similar emotions or rubrics. Take into account various rubrics that express the same feelings to avoid skewing your case towards one remedy. For example, the rubrics—*ailments from grief, from disappointed love, from anger, from masturbation,* and *from rudeness*—may all belong to one layer and, in fact, all belong to one remedy, *Staphysagria*! This is not surprising since most remedies have different causalities in their proving symptoms. Please don't follow the advice of some schools that, "You can only choose one NWS." Not if they all belong to the same layer! Why would you consider only one NWS when others were responsible for the creation of the delusions and compensations of the patient? That would make no sense at all!

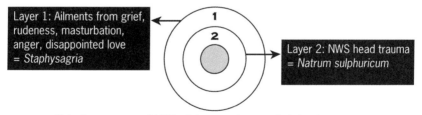

FINDING THE SIMILLIMUM

Layer 1: Ailments from grief, rudeness, masturbation, anger, disappointed love = *Staphysagria*

Layer 2: NWS head trauma = *Natrum sulphuricum*

Take into account all NWS of the same layer to find the simillimum!

Of course, homeopathy, more than any other modality, will try to detect an emotional causality rather than a physical one. Among women, delusions created by severe fixed emotions (a painful, repressed complex according to Carl Jung) are often most linked to affairs of the heart (whether perceived or real): deception, lack of love, loss of love, unrequited love, etc. With men, we most likely find that delusions are formed relative to business affairs, image, and prestige: the sword-wielding man is more interested in conquering land and becoming famous than in shielding his heart.

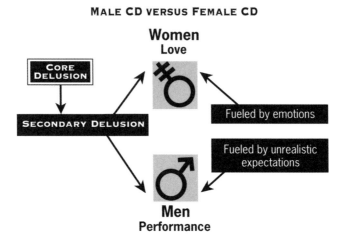

MALE CD VERSUS FEMALE CD

Searching for the NWS: A Difficult Task

Never underestimate how far back in the patient's history the homeopath must go (even back to intrauterine events). The homeopath should never be surprised to find identical triggers in various layers of the same case as humans tend to fall down a lot before they learn their lesson or to sink back into situations that are familiar to them, no matter how terrible. More unfortunately, some patients are subjected to a repeated strong emotion (the Chinese would call this "noble misfortunes" in comparison with those we impose on ourselves, which they call "ignoble") such as fright, which then creates a core delusion responsible for the patient's behavior. Repetition of a situation, such as repeated ailments from fright, is linked to a core delusion that the patient becomes enslaved to (see Chap. 6).

An example of the repetition of such "noble misfortune" was displayed in a young boy who had "behavioral problems" at school and at home. His behavior at home included losing his temper, hitting, maliciousness, intolerance of contradiction, hateful speech, cruel treatment of animals, and low self-esteem. These behaviors stood in contrast to his school behavior where he was taciturn, crying when he made mistakes, demonstrating silliness and foolishness while letting himself be abused by others. He didn't stand up for himself because he "wanted everyone to be his friend."

This child was diagnosed with the newest fad in allopathy, "Selective Mutism," but to the astute homeopath, such a "split personality" is quite familiar.

Looking for possible causalities, I went back to the pregnancy to discover if the mother had suffered possible emotional traumas, which would have been transmitted to the unborn fetus. The mother was alone when pregnant because her husband was traveling all the time. She felt forsaken **and** fearful: "What if something happens to me? I am all alone here." And when her husband was at home, he worked very late: "I never got his attention!" These facts evoked strong feelings of anger and irritability in the mother, and all these emotions were carried over to the fetus, the best proof seen in that child's present behavior. This emotional rejection almost resulted in a physical one when the mother suffered from eclampsia in her third trimester. I knew I needed a "fright- and anger-filled remedy" to resolve the child's case.

This 12-year-old child's strong "Jekyll and Hyde" behavior was caused by a later repetition of the emotions experienced as a fetus. When the child was two, the mom locked herself out on the balcony by accident. Separated by the glass door, she saw her son going into a complete melt-down of hysterical screaming and crying. When the firemen came and picked the child up, he screamed in terror as he saw this as further separation from his mom, frightening him even more. This was a second event in which the child experienced terror, fright, and the feeling of being forsaken.

A third trauma was the birth of a younger sister. Although he initially reacted lovingly to the baby, his behavior had already changed by the time the baby was 14 days old. He now appeared to be jealous of his sister, demonstrating extreme sexual behavior towards both parents. For the homeopath, this evokes a delusion of *Hyoscyamus, is going to be sold*, which can be linked to fear of abandonment. The homeopath can easily link the three traumas together and find the simillimum for this case (*Hyoscyamus*).

Most patients will surprise you with an exact memory of whatever the trigger may be; the exact time and date are often recalled. That, of course, leaves out those patients who, as compensation, repress their NWS. This blank state of mind is an act of self-defense as evidenced in the orphan who may require *Magnesium carbonicum*. Why remember things from the past that are too painful? For instance, say the NWS was heartbreak: the patient grew up with two alcoholic parents, effectively making him an orphan. "I have to move on," he says. "I can't afford to dwell on this. I don't want to go there. I already resolved that issue!" Of course he did not; he is a major work in progress! People who suppress their emotions are initially equally reluctant to discuss their NWS, even if they remember it. The reason is self-protection: better to be over-cautious than get burnt yet again! As much as these characters hide their NWS, consciously or unconsciously, what they can't hide is how they are dealing with it. The homeopath can work his way back through Aphorism 153 rubrics and fixed ideas (compensations) to find the patient's secret NWS in order to treat him. Don't make the mistake of linking the entire progress of the patient to the remedy's action. One of my students, a great mom, was so excited to see a change in her teenager's behavior that she exclaimed, "The remedy is working." This enraged the teenager because it did not take into account her own psychological problem. Better to observe and give support when asked!

Sometimes the mother of the child/children you are treating has died, and you can't get the intrauterine story from the father, who often regards such information as nonsense, especially if the trigger (the "crime") points to him. Don't insist and make yourself an enemy! Through the rest of the information (not least, by carefully observing the behavior of the child), you can find out what most likely happened. If you do, keep it to yourself instead of playing the know-it-all and judge.

Often, NWS information is missing because a child is adopted and by law, nothing—not even the medical history of the birth parents—is known. While this is unfortunate, the homeopath still can find the simillimum. It is like a puzzle of 100 pieces where one important piece is missing: fitting together the rest of the pieces shows you the end icture anyway.

I can cite here a beautiful example where the adoptive mother of the patient could not recall the NWS and was in fact absolutely unaware of it (the rubrics I chose are in italics).

This was the case of an adopted child who exhibited reckless and foolish behavior. I saw him when he was 6 years old, and the adoptive parent told me:

> He dances like a monkey to music (*foolish behavior; sensitive;* and *music ameliorates*); he is impulsive and cannot sit still unless he's watching TV (*restlessness while sitting*). He does not like contradiction (*intolerant of contradiction*) and annoys people to the point of being malicious (*maliciousness*). He never obeys me. When he plays outside, I have to go get him and literally pull him into the house (*disobedience*). What worries me though is that he will talk to any stranger, such as workers in the street (*amativeness*). He often *refuses to answer* or gives an answer totally unrelated to the question. He acts the same way at school. He is cruel (*malicious; cruelty*) to our blind dog, hits him or jumps on him. He tells lies about his older sister, 'she is mean, teaches me bad words, and offends me.' Of course he does this when he is caught saying bad words (*cunning*).

All this fixed behavior could be traced back to the boy's birth mother. She became pregnant with her second child so that her boyfriend would marry her! The first child was adopted by the same family (the older sister mentioned above) but was a totally normal and affectionate child! Luckily for me, the adoptive mother knew the story of the birth mother, an exception!

So both are children of the same biological parents, yet they are 100 percent different. Why? The birth parents had decided early in the pregnancy to put the first child up for adoption, so there were no negative feelings. However, in the case of the second child, having become pregnant with the intent of forcing her boyfriend to marry her, the birth mother only decided to put the child up for adoption two weeks before delivery, after her boyfriend stood firm on his decision not to keep this baby either!

A situation, called "*ailments from unrequited love*," had been transmitted to this unfortunate child in the intrauterine environment, and he now showed all the symptoms of *Tarentula*, which was in fact his simillimum. The typical triad of symptoms for *Tarentula*—cunning, restless, and mischievous—is easily seen in this boy's case.

Question 8: What is the Core Delusion?

The Birth of Delusions and the Core Delusion

The highest value among Aphorism 153 symptoms is accorded to delusions (see Chap. 9, *Hahnemann Revisited*). Delusions or fixed ideas are created by unresolved, long-lasting, painful events. Delusions always contain a kernel of truth. As mentioned before, in the case of males, delusions often have to do with performance, work, achievements, and standing in society. In women, delusions are most often linked to affairs of the heart: loss of love, perceived or real; unrequited love; deception; betrayal, etc. For example, the woman is usually the one who tells her husband, "You forgot my birthday today," not a very important event for him, and one he is likely to forget. Many of our delusions stem from unrealistic and exaggerated expectations. Delusions are created by aiming for things that are out of our reach, by underestimating difficulties, by having unjustified optimism, or by being overly anxious, jealous, greedy, egotistical, etc.

Among all the patient's presenting delusions, **one** started the whole process: the core delusion (CD)—the primal, archaic, or original delusion. The CD is the source of all subsequent delusions or fixed ideas, which are created because the patient received inadequate support or therapy. The CD is the center point or nucleus, the beginning of the patient's story, and it indicates the remedy he needs! Therefore, discovering the CD will be an important step, not only in formulating and understanding the crux of the patient's suffering, but also in finding the similar remedy that will free him from the chains of his central, fixed idea. In addition, the CD will help the homeopath differentiate between two or three remedies at the end of the consultation. The correct interpretation of the CD must match the secondary delusions and their compensations through provings of the remedy, the **only** standard we apply in homeopathy to separate truth from fiction. (I typically refer to the provings of Hahnemann, Hering, and T. F. Allen.) When looking at the totality of symptoms, the CD cannot be taken out of the context (see Aphorisms 5 and 7). The CD expresses the most important characteristic of the patient's totality. This has prompted me to formulate another definition of the CD. *The CD is the emotional or spiritual center, surrounded by a cluster of images or ideas which are the patient's compensations.*

How shall we further define the CD? How can we identify it?

IDENTIFYING THE CORE DELUSION

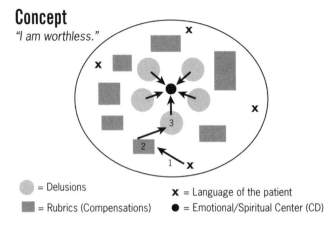

Concept

"I am worthless."

= Delusions   **x** = Language of the patient

= Rubrics (Compensations)   ● = Emotional/Spiritual Center (CD)

Defining Core Delusions and Compensations

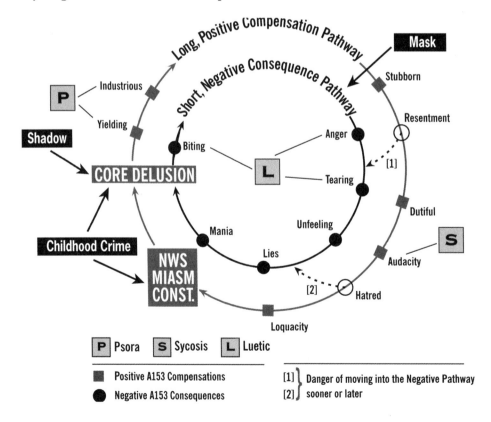

P Psora   **S** Sycosis   **L** Luetic

■ Positive A153 Compensations

● Negative A153 Consequences

[1] } Danger of moving into the Negative Pathway
[2] } sooner or later

The CD is *the expression of the dominant, ruling emotion*. It drives the actions, thoughts, and plans of the patient, creating, along the way, *secondary* delusions. For example, *Lachesis* has the CD that *he is injured by his surroundings; that he is wronged*. When this situation is persistent (as it **is** by definition in the case of a delusion), it will lead inevitably to secondary delusions such as: *he will be sent to an asylum* and *his medicine is poison*. These are expressions of a paranoid delusional state, proof of further evolving pathology often ending in schizophrenia. Thus, all compensations and secondary delusions have their origin in the CD. For example, a patient needing *Lachesis* might be loquacious, have religious fixations, meditate, and have increased sexual activity. It is imperative for everyone (as we *all* have a CD) to effect compensations, which can be regarded as *defense mechanisms* aimed at fleeing from a negative CD or reinforcing a positive CD. The patient may create lots of compensations to avoid his fate, yet ultimately, he will have to face this CD at some point in his life. Even a "good" delusion such as, *humility of others while he is great* (*Platina, Staphysagria*), is obviously bad for the person as it reflects a delusion of grandeur and impedes self-growth. If "positive" psoric compensations persist, over time their intensity will grow excessive (sycosis) and ultimately become destructive (syphilitic or luetic) to others and the self.

One of my best students, Rachele Mazza-Aives, expressed the CD beautifully: *the CD is the one fixed idea that guides my every move*. Dr. von Boenninghausen's use of the following questions clarifies what Rachele said (*Lesser Writings of von Boenninghausen*, pp. 105-112). The CD tells me:

How (*Quomodo*)?	To react, to feel, to act
What (*Quid*)?	To eat, to wear, to do or not do, to say
Where (*Ubi*)?	To find solace, comfort, and stimulation
When (*Quando*)?	Is my best/worst time of the day; when do I peak or drop?
Who (*Quis*)?	Who do I bring into my inner circle? Whom can I trust? Who am I? What is my Persona?
With What (*Quibus auxillis*)?	Can I achieve my goals? What are my tools?
Why (*Cur*)?	Am I acting this way? Why do I think this way?

The same questions can be asked to determine the predominant miasmatic state of the patient, which demonstrates the close relationship between the predominant miasm and the CD.

The Five Why's: Confirming the Core Delusion

We must try to answer the question: How do we find the expression or compensation closest to the CD or better still, one that directly expresses the CD? How do we avoid prescribing based on compensations (Persona or mask) far removed from the CD? Once we have found, or think we have found, the CD or a compensation close to the CD, it is important to make sure that it is the *basic* or *primary* delusion by asking one more WHY, if at all possible.

At a conference, one of my students heard the speaker suggesting that in any behavioral situation one should ask oneself "why" five times, each time working from the previous answer. By the fifth "why," a hint of the emotional state of affairs that underlies the feeling or situation will become evident. While it might be arbitrary to ask "why" five times, at least by concentrating on five, the homeopath will not stop questioning too early when assessing his patient. If the patient decided to go back to an ex-boyfriend, for example, this might at first sound like reconciliation, a positive step, which would not be taken into account in finding the simillimum. Upon further questioning, however, the homeopath finds out that the patient did return not because she thought breaking up was a mistake or because she still loved the old boyfriend; instead, the homeopath finds that the patient wants to go back because she felt lonely and craves attention (possibly indicating the remedy *Pulsatilla*). Or maybe the motivation was to exact revenge: to make up simply in order to break up the relationship herself, to "have the last word," so to speak (a classic response in the case of *Aurum*). Or suppose someone wants to go to graduate school, not because he wants to get ahead in life through education but simply to earn the respect and love of his family, which he so much desires. Here, after one more "why," the delusion, *I am not loved*, may become the delusion, *I am worthless*, and thus transform itself into the delusion, *I never succeed in anything* (*Aurum muriaticum natronatum, Argentum nitricum, Anacardium, Baryta carbonica*). If the answer to the next "why" is: "Because everyone criticizes me," then we have the delusion criticized, which is a fixed idea that is not at all typical of the above-mentioned remedies. If you then asked the question, "How do you feel about this?" in order to elicit the ruling emotion and thus the CD, the patient might answer, "I feel like a cripple and cannot make any decisions." This statement can be translated into the delusions: *he walks on his knees; his legs are cut off*. And that answer would confirm a prescription of *Baryta carbonica*. If, at this point, no further "why" can be asked, we can safely assume that we have arrived at the patient's CD, one belonging to *Baryta carbonica*.

Although this person thinks getting a degree will be the road to self worth, he does not know that he has simply relegated his delusion that he is not loved to the unconscious where it awaits its next opportunity to return.

If we don't ask a sufficient number of "why's," the patient will show us compensations far removed from their CD. We will then be prescribing for the mask rather than the shadow side—the mask formed by all these compensations. This will lead to the selection of a simile, for:

The mask is the simile; the shadow side is the simillimum!

An ancient Chinese proverb expresses the same:

> Confucius says: To return to the root (CD!) is to find the meaning, but to pursue appearance (compensations!) is to miss the source!

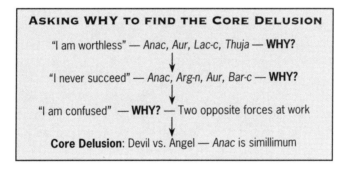

Take for example a patient who says, "I am worthless." On first consideration, this *is* an Aphorism 153 symptom and can be used to find the simillimum. At this point, the homeopath might consider remedies like *Anacardium*, *Aurum*, *Lac caninum*, and *Thuja*. In fact, however, we need to ask "Why do you feel this way?" in order to find an Aphorism 153 symptom that more closely describes the shadow side or CD. That will help us make a differential diagnosis among the previously mentioned remedies. The patient might answer, "Because I never succeed with anything" (delusions: *he does everything wrong; he can not succeed*— see *Anacardium, Argentum nitricum, Aurum, Baryta carbonica*). If we stop here, it appears that *Aurum* and *Anacardium* are in the running, being present in both rubrics. On the next "why" the patient might reply, "Because I am confused, since there are two opposite forces at work, and I can't make up my mind. Sometimes I get into trouble because of my decisions. It is as if there are two persons in me with two different opinions. One voice seems to tell me to do my business fast, even in a dishonest way, since it will bring me more profit. At the same time, the other voice, I guess my conscience, tells me to be honest and serve people rather than take advantage of them. And I never really know who is going to win: my conscience or the dishonest voice."

Finally we have come to the CD—the crux of this patient's suffering. He suffers from the delusion that *a devil is speaking in one ear prompting to murder, and an angel in the other ear, prompting to acts of benevolence.* This symptom belongs to *Anacardium* and is often caused by *ailments from domination* during childhood.

Triggers Leading to the Core Delusion

The painful event leading to the birth of the CD is most often of a mental/ emotional nature: death of loved one; betrayal; discovering as a teenager that your father had an affair; indignation; rudeness; domination, etc. However, a *physical illness* like pneumonia also can cause the onset of a delusion. For example, a case of pneumonia leading to chronic fatigue can change the patient into a person with low energy and great lack of self-confidence. He now has the delusion, *he cannot succeed in anything,* even though after some time, his physical energy returns. The pneumonia has left a "scar" on more than just the physical plane, a scar which has undermined his self-confidence. This happens even more frequently in patients who have suffered a heart attack or stroke: the patient now has the delusion *that he is about to die,* causing him to feel he is a lesser person than he was before. Clearing this delusion will require *Aconite.* Or the patient may claim, "I caught pneumonia because I smoked eight cigarettes a day for several months years ago," which would refer to the fixed idea that he *has ruined his health* (*Chelidonium*).

Another example could be a person with Chronic Fatigue and Immune Dysfunction Syndrome (CFIDS), expressed through various liver and gallbladder problems. Because of her disease, this previously vibrant person now feels totally isolated to the point of thinking *she has no friends.* Here we all recognize the syphilitic phase of *Magnesium muriaticum,* the peacemaker in the household and in his environment, who will yield to others at the expense of his own wishes and emotions.

Let's look at a brief summation of such an example from the practice. A 30-year-old woman comes for a consult. Both parents smoked marijuana when her mother was pregnant with her. After a few years, the patient's mother divorced the father to whom the patient was close (*homesickness*), and now mother remarries an alcoholic who tortures the daughter emotionally and physically (ailments from *domination*; delusion, *someone walks behind him*). This someone is not a friendly guide, but rather a negative controlling person. The mother also becomes an alcoholic. We can well imagine that at that time the child must have felt alone (delusions: *all alone in the world*; *she is friendless*).

The patient starts smoking marijuana almost daily from age 12 on (presumably in order to escape into a dream world to avoid her pain, as she also tried to commit suicide by cutting her veins—*anguish, loathing, homesickness*—expressing the syphilitic taint). She marries a kind man but during her pregnancy she is hospitalized with a serious liver problem resulting in much fear and depression (*fear, in affections of the liver*). Although the liver problem has improved, she now suffers from depression for which she takes allopathic drugs and undergoes psychotherapy.

After beginning therapy, she loses her memory for past events. She "wants everyone to like her" (CD: *she is friendless!*; *sadness when alone*); she will do whatever it takes to obtain love and affection. She can't stand it when people don't get along, and she feels it is *her* duty to bring peace. She is bitter because most of the time when she helps someone, she is condemned for it (*discouraged*). Everyone must be happy, even when achieving that state brings her suffering and humiliation; she cannot say no. If people dislike each other, she agonizes over what she could do to restore peace. Sometimes her mind speaks with two voices (*confusion of mind*).

Treatment: 1 pellet of *Magnesium muriaticum* 1M in an 8-oz. Remedy Stock Bottle (RSB), 1 succussion, dilute 1 tsp. in a 4-oz. cup of purified water, take 1 tsp. as a test dose.

Result: Two days later she is full of energy, cleaning the house, and throwing old things out. Her husband remarks that he hasn't seen her so energetic in a long time. She notices that she can now more easily express her opinion in the therapy group at the hospital. She is feeling so good that she even starts fearing that her doctors will terminate her therapy sessions (she likes attending therapy and talking about her childhood with others). She feels like she has been drinking 20 cups of coffee a day. Interestingly, her need for sweets has disappeared, too! (She is overweight because of all that sugar.)

Three days later: The need for sweets returned yesterday. And her energy level is falling. Add 1 succussion to the RSB and repeat the remedy.

Report: The remedy didn't work as fantastically as the first dose. The need for sweets remained. A 4-oz. RSB of *Magnesium muriaticum* 1M is prepared and 2 succussions are added to the RSB (i.e., succussions added are equivalent to the ones added to the first 8-oz. RSB). This patient has a strong Vital Force (VF) and no aggravation or accessory symptoms occurred. This indicates that the patient can tolerate a stronger potency. Thus the homeopath can switch from an 8-oz. RSB to a 4-oz. RSB.

On the morning of following day, the patient adds 2 succussions to the 4-oz. RSB, dilutes 1 tsp. in 4 oz. of purified water and takes 1 tsp. from the 4-oz. cup.

Next day: The remedy has worked again! No desire for sweets. She begins to feel heat in the face.

Three days later: The remedy is fading out again. Repeat the remedy every three days, adding 4 succussions each time!

The only "ill effect" to be mentioned: she got a cold after the first dose, with a lot of discharge from the lungs, but she says she gets this every winter, so it is not unusual. For me, this also indicates an "exteriorization and healing reaction," an action of the VF (Aphorism 64).

Other physical causalities that come to mind are car accidents, maybe leading to disfigurement and thus creating the delusions: *wretched when looking in the mirror* (*Natrum muriaticum*); *he is short; he is diminished; he is hideous and distorted.* A person needing *Lac caninum* as can develop these delusions from a situation where someone is treated badly by a "wicked stepmother."

How to Find the Core Delusion in the Clinic

The whole of our investigation is geared toward finding the core or "mother" delusion. Yet you cannot expect to receive an answer from your patient if you phrase your question: "What is your core delusion?" He won't just come to you and offer the information, "Doctor, I have the basic delusion that I am a bottle!" How then do we go about determining the CD?

A first hint of the CD can be found by paying attention to the manner in which the patient **communicates** with you. It is interesting how patients who have strong delusions have a tendency to speak in *absolutes*, using words like "*always, never, everybody, nobody, all or nothing.*" Their perception of the world seems to count for everyone at any time. For people with delusions, there are no shades of gray. Everything is black or white. There is no flexibility, just opinions cast in stone that form the guidelines according to which life evolves, to that person's way of thinking. Such speaking in absolutes indicates fixed ideas. Pay attention to where the patient uses these absolutes: these moments point to the CD.

A second hint is that during live case-taking, the patient often *betrays the CD* when a very painful issue is touched upon, by even as so much as a small hint, reference, or thought. The CD is always linked to a painful, unresolved complex from the past that was allowed to grow to the extent that the patient is now addicted to it. It is the "baggage" that the patient carries around and brings along into any relationship, and that baggage has become an integral part of the patient. Such a "high feeling complex" is easily touched upon, even obliquely, by an innocent word or question. A *"complex" is a picture—often of a psychologically traumatic or painful nature—that has become part of the contents of the unconscious.* It constitutes the personal and private side of psychic life, therefore, it is often suppressed (the *Natrums*) or repressed (the *Magnesiums*).

Whenever the homeopath touches on such a delicate complex, the patient may react with telltale **indicators** such as silence, anger, irritability, crying, subsequent failure to remember the response, hesitation, lengthened response time, or stuttering. The patient may even close her eyes for an instant. **Suppression:** the patient feels the emotions and then suppresses them! **Repression:** the patient does not even feel the emotions. Repression is stronger than suppression.

When this happens, the homeopath must realize that his words or gestures have evoked a painful Never Well Since (NWS) event in the patient's homeopathic history. Let it sink in, let the patient cry, and meanwhile, focus silently on what you just have touched upon. For example, the mother of a physically or mentally "challenged" child responds in the consultation when you discuss her pregnancy. Does she feel guilty because when she heard she was pregnant, she "really did not want that child," for whatever reason? Was it because you touched her "Achilles heel," and the memory of a suppressed grief, the real cause of onset of her physical problem, is brought to the surface? Many times, in probing gently for the "scene of the crime," I have discovered the painful concept that gave rise to the CD. (I refer the reader also to my "11 case-taking questions," see p. 5). Remember to be compassionate in your inquiry! You don't want to be perceived as a prosecutor on a fact-finding mission, even though we talk about the NWS as "the scene of the crime!"

The third way to recognize when you've touch on the CD of your patient occurs when he is forced to approach a situation with his inferior function of consciousness (see Chap. 10)! This rule is as follows:

The negative CD appears strongly when someone is forced to operate with his inferior function of consciousness. This person will try to make the CD disappear through the positive compensations available to him. The positive CD is supported by the dominant function of consciousness *and* his positive compensations.

As we can see, positive compensations are used for an entirely opposite goal than in the instance concerning the negative CD. Let's explain this with an example.

—

One example of the first rule (appearance of a negative CD) is *Lycopodium*, predominantly a thinking person. As long as he can hide behind his superior function (thought processes), he is in control of his actions, but when he is forced to approach a situation with his feelings, he loses control and resorts to childish behavior. At that point, his CD, *he has done wrong and everything will disappear*, bursts forth with great intensity.

An example of the "positive" delusion is the CD of *Ignatia: she is married and pregnant. Ignatia* is predominantly a feeling person. If she is forced to operate on the thinking and reasoning plane, her positive delusion dissolves! *Ignatia* has put so much of her emotional baggage into a relationship that an insignificant remark by the object of her desire such as "you're looking nice today" may be construed as a powerful and objective proof of his love. The slightest hint of appreciation is incorporated into the delusion and elaborated with complete blindness to even the weightiest arguments to the contrary. It is only when she remains in her feeling function that she can maintain this CD through her positive compensations: romantic, sentimental, finely sensitive mood, mild, and quiet disposition. She bears suffering without outrage or complaint; thinking about the loved one ameliorates.

More Tools for Finding the Core Delusion During the Consult

The Ruling Emotion

Sometimes in the interview, the patient will directly admit to his *ruling emotion*: "I feel I don't fit in this world!" Other times, this same dominant emotion (as mentioned above, *the feeling of being forsaken*) will be expressed during the initial interview with the patient, when he answers various questions (see example in Chap. 5 in the section "Searching for the NWS: A Difficult Task"). Although the patient will use different words and speak of various situations, they all express the feeling of being forsaken. It may start with the patient's *intrauterine history* where his mother suffered a "forsaken" incident, then continue with lack of emotional nourishment from the parents, followed by failed relationships; the death of close friends; betrayal by spouse; isolation at work; or sense of isolation because of a handicap, language barrier, cultural differences, etc. No matter how thick the presenting patient's mask is, the ruling emotion manages to leak through when the homeopath asks himself: "What sense, what dominant emotion, do I get from this patient?"

The homeopath must be able to zoom in on this dominant emotion. Homeopaths have a great **power of observation**, which can be helpful to solve this riddle. I remember how some patients sit in front of me and talk in exaggerated, hysterical tones about a multitude of ailments, and even more frequently, about trifles like, "Why does my tan line not fade sooner?" and "Why is this one nail not growing as fast as the others?" Their painful expression and their hurried loquacity confirm that the patient views these "imperfections" as life-threatening or as direct expressions of a failing health (delusions: *suffers from an incurable disease; he is sick*).

Besides observation and careful attention to what the patient expresses indirectly, we can resort to **directly questioning** the patient. This type of questioning is helpful only with an intelligent patient, one who absolutely wants to get better and who can be honest with you, the homeopath. Ask directly, "What is your strongest negative emotion? What is your strongest positive emotion? What emotion 'rules' you?" To my surprise, patients can often easily tell me what their all-consuming emotion was or is: grief, jealousy, anxiety for the future, lack of self-worth, financial concerns, lack of direction and meaning in life, etc. If the patient does not manage to express his all-consuming emotion, ask the spouse!

One of the best techniques to identify delusions in the clinic is a general discussion with the patient: about his work, politics, the world, family, friends, his childhood, vacations, etc. This is especially the case with that class of patients who are secretive or ashamed of certain aspects in their past, or someone who is forced to come to see you by their spouse, or the unruly teenager who does not want to see this special doctor who asks probing questions. During the discussion, observe how the patient thinks and how he expresses himself. By having empathy for the patient, you will make him feel at ease, and he may be able to express his deepest feelings to you, even unconsciously. In this way, you gain precious information to use in finding the simillimum.

A beautiful example of this from my practice was a patient who did not want to see me. He arrived in a black suit with a big cross hanging on his chest, and I immediately asked him to tell me about his "mission." I never had to ask another question. He opened up to me about his delusion of "being in communication with God." His feeling that he must spread the word of God (*delusion, he is in heaven talking with God; Veratrum album* is graded a 2 and is the only remedy in the rubric) and save the souls of prostitutes and homeless people in Los Angeles became immediately apparent. He was driven by a strong desire to "be somebody," which we translate into the rubric, *despair of social position*. Yet to the initial question, "What can I do for you?" he had answered, "There's nothing the matter with me; my wife brought me here." Of course, he did not tell me that he had been banned from every church for interrupting services to give his own sermon, or that he became violent when contradicted while *squandering the family's money* (*Veratrum album*). This applied technique might be called finding the CD through "indirect" questioning.

The dominant emotion is intrinsically linked to the NWS. It sometimes happens that the patient cannot recall the NWS or an important emotional event. For example, *Carbon* people in general concentrate on the slightest physical ailments and fail to make any connection with psychological triggers. While *Carbons* don't do this intentionally, others, like the *Natrums*, view questions about their private emotional life as overbearing and intruding; only when you gain their trust will they confide their most intimate details which have been suppressed for a long time. The *Magnesium* personality, on the other hand, has not **su**ppressed but **re**pressed her emotions: these sensations are not even felt for a moment, but the *Magnesiums* are not conscious of what they are concealing. It must be mentioned that if we are conscious of what we are hiding (like the *Natrums*), decidedly less harm is done than if we do not know what we are repressing (the *Magnesiums*), or worse still, if we don't know that we have repressed anything at all. Suppressed and repressed emotions are often linked to a secret, something not allowed to surface because it is too painful or too shameful to recall. These emotions become part of our unconscious world, our shadow side, stored away safely but ready to leave Pandora's box when home-opathic remedies or psychoanalysis open the door to the unconscious world. This can happen through a trigger, some event or word or gesture that alludes to that stored, fixed, painful, or shameful emotion or delusion, which at that point may come crashing into the consciousness of the patient! Locking away and holding back emotions is a *psychic mistake* for which nature will compensate by creating physical illness.

It is easy to understand why *Magnesium carbonicum* represses his emotions: he has had a life like that of an orphan (*dreams, lost in the forest and lost at home*) and needs all his practical senses to get through each day. Emotions are to him only a hindrance, distracting him and clouding the sense of practical street wisdom he needs to survive and to obtain his most basic needs. In spite of controlling their feelings marvelously well, such patients can be terribly bothered by them, as is shown by their *irritability* and their severe spastic pains everywhere, with diarrhea and cutting pain. I wonder how many so-called "fibromyalgia" patients have such roots in their history! The *Magnesium muriaticum* person is the unfortunate one caught up in losing an existing relationship (to parents, siblings, or friends) and who will therefore do anything, especially repress his own feelings (as does a *Carcinosin*) to make peace (*delusion, he is friendless*) and assure the relationship.

An example would be a child trying to intervene between two quarreling parents who are contemplating divorce. The physical results can be terrible as this repression can result in liver and gallbladder symptoms as well as CFIDS (see the *Magnesium muriaticum* example above).

The attitude and professionalism of the homeopath will also play a role in uncovering the patient's dominant emotion. Being an empathetic, attentive homeopath is a must. The practice of any art and science requires **discipline**, and the homeopath must regularly study his science. Self-discipline is hard to come by nowadays as the modern person, outside of his routine job, often just wants to be lazy. As always, good practice also requires an absolutely perfect inquiry, that is, case-taking done to the best of our ability. **Concentration** is another must and rather rare in our culture. Far too often, the homeopath is distracted by everyday problems that have nothing to do with the patient in front of him. **Patience,** another necessity, may be the biggest obstacle of all. Driven by the consumer's demand for fast results, availability of other modalities, and hollow promises of speedy relief, homeopaths make most of their case-management mistakes by not waiting long enough for the VF to respond to the simillimum.

For some homeopaths, **intuition** is a very natural thing, allowing them to understand aspects of the patient intuitively before they register them intellectually. This intuition makes up for what one cannot perceive or think or feel and is therefore greatly needed by a good homeopath or indeed by any doctor. Many good insights come from this very mysterious function.

Last but not least, the highest quality of any healer is **humility**. To be objective and non-judgmental, one has to be humble—the emotional attitude behind reason. Emotional attitude and reason are indivisible!

Not a Method for Physical Problems?

Asking "What is the dominant emotion?" makes it appear that this is not a method for determining treatment for physical complaints but rather one limited to cases where mental/emotional symptoms predominate. The homeopath must remember that most chronic physical problems also have a mental/emotional issue at their onset or as causality. An example of this would be a history of chronic headache or migraine, where the problem began simultaneously with a divorce. Or we find chronic backaches in a woman caught up in an unhealthy relationship (e.g., *Natrum muriaticum, Sepia*). Here too, we must inform ourselves concerning the basic feelings and reactions of the patient. What physical problem did the patients' emotions create?

"Physical suffering" and expressions originating in emotions were very clear in yet another patient's story. She took four days off at the seashore by herself, swam, walked, and was amazed that her sciatica, stiff joints, and nasal discharge disappeared during that time. Coming home to the husband who had deceived her in the past immediately opened the floodgates to her physical symptoms. Not surprisingly, in view of the strong amelioration at the seashore and ailments from deception and betrayal, *Natrum muriaticum* was the simillimum. Better yet, the patient was obliged to acknowledge the causality between her physical suffering and the emotions triggered by her negative emotional environment. On the other hand, when chronic headaches stem from head trauma experienced in a car accident, this CD method should not be applied; a von Boenninghausen analysis might be a more logical approach in that case.

Another example of delusions related to negative emotional events that resulted in physical expressions was the case of a three-year-old girl who had a crop of warts on the back of her hand. These warts made their appearance shortly after the death of her grandfather of whom she was very fond and whom she would visit every day! After his death, she stopped drawing, something she loved to do, for more than eight months (*delusion, alone, being: always alone; she is*)! The grief apparently awoke in her a latent sycotic miasm with a wart expression. So a sycotic grief remedy was needed and not *Thuja*!

Aphorism 153 Symptoms

In many cases, neither the NWS nor the ruling emotion is known to the patient. How do we proceed then? Begin with a blank image of the pathways of delusions (see "Pathways of the Delusions" figure on p. 48). This is the background or **blueprint** on which you will put together your puzzle, the patient!

Every intense and peculiar symptom found in the patient and matched in the same intensity to the remedy will represent an important piece of the patient's puzzle. We can now work backwards on this blueprint. As various pieces of the puzzle are put together, the picture of two or three close remedies may evolve. Look at the delusions of these remedies to determine what set of delusions (or if you know it, which CD) best fits the patient's case. One of the easiest ways to become familiar with the meaning of delusions is by watching live cases. A live-patient case clarifies better than anything else the meaning of a delusion.

If the patient cannot recall the NWS, the physician must proceed with a series of "why and for what purpose" questions concerning the most peculiar **Aphorism 153 mental and emotional** characteristics of the patient, since these will bring forth the CD. (The NWS is always superior to the Aphorism 153 symptoms, as explained in *Hahnemann Revisited*). Strange, rare, and peculiar can also be of a physical nature, for instance, the association of coryza and perspiration in the remedy *Mercurius*. In general, when using the CD method, the homeopath will limit himself to the mental/emotional Aphorism 153 rubrics. We will be especially interested in those Aphorism 153 rubrics that Carl Jung refers to as emotions, rather than feelings. I agree with the distinction he makes between these two: emotions rule us; feelings are less passionate.

In French, the word "*sentiment*" signifies both "feeling" and "opinion." For example, "It is the *sentiment* of the Principal that ..." When you have feelings— especially in the case of those that lack an emotional element, for example, feeling at peace, feeling content, feeling serene and in balance—you are still in control. Emotions affect and possibly rule you. The emotions of others also affect you, for example, when you are in an enthusiastic crowd watching a soccer match. Most of us cannot avoid being caught up in the momentary contagion of the crowd's jubilant emotion. I remember standing at a Euro 2000 soccer match in Belgium, in the midst of Spaniards and Yugoslavians, as it was a match between Yugoslavia and Spain. Being a Belgian, I had no favorite; I just hoped to attend a great match. Yet, when the Yugoslavian team scored a goal, I found myself dancing in triumph with a Yugoslavian supporter—not because I wanted Yugoslavia to win, but simply because I was caught up in the burst of joy and hilarity! Then Spain made a goal, and I found myself dancing in the arms of a Spanish supporter. Am I a traitor? No! I am overcome and inspired by the emotion around me.

As you can see, it really is a question of degree: "emotion" evokes stronger physiological reactions (pulse, respiration) than does a "feeling." You could call a "feeling" the precursor of "emotion" in instances when some psychic control is lost. To us homeopaths, once we have gathered enough of those true, intensely Aphorism 153 emotional rubrics, the most persistent and deepest emotions, the ruling emotion—often repressed in the CD—becomes clear.

Here is an example. The patient was betrayed by a lover but does not want to tell you about it, thinking it has no bearing on his chief complaint, twitching leg muscles. On the other hand, he uses lewd language, talks of sexual desire, is easily enraged and, in this state of rage, may try to kill someone, usually with a knife. Yet he desires company and has fear of being alone, so you might think of *Hyoscyamus*. When studying *Hyoscyamus*, we find delusions of *being sold, being injured by his surroundings*, and *he has suffered wrong*. If these delusions fit the totality of the case, we are led to the patient's NWS, oftentimes ailments from *grief and disappointed love with great jealousy* in the case of *Hyoscyamus*. As one can see, we always ask ourselves: "Do these Aphorism 153 rubrics fit the perceived delusion?" If so, we can uncover the patient's CD, confirming his simillimum. Discovering the vicious cycle the patient has fallen prey to and explaining it to the patient in an empathetic way will accelerate his evolution in a very positive direction. Also see the *Tarentula* case example at the end of Chapter 5.

The following case shows how the practitioner can work backwards. During one of my teaching breaks, a student of mine asked me to help him gain some insight into a case. I had just taught how one must look at compensating Aphorism 153 symptoms and try to work backwards, if necessary to the intrauterine period, to find the real CD with the help of the NWS.

The following is the story of a four-year-old boy with a morbidly intense need for affection and attention. Remedies such as *Pulsatilla* and *Hyoscyamus* immediately come to mind, but he exhibited neither violent nor sexual behavior, nor lewd talk, nor even jealousy. The boy had a younger sister and if anything, he was very concerned for her safety, always looking after her (*sympathetic; anxiety for others*). That certainly eliminated *Hyoscyamus*. *Pulsatilla* became doubtful when I heard that, not only was he not jealous of his sister but he had had no difficulties going to school for the first time. In fact, when his mom waited at the doorway, he told her "to go on home, that he was OK"—and indeed he was.

At home he could play for hours by himself and did not need anyone else. *Pulsatilla* just did not seem to fit. Other symptoms he displayed were: easily angered, sensitive to admonition (a sycotic trait), *antagonistic toward himself*, low self-esteem ("I am dumb") even to the point of asking for punishment. He spoke eloquently (indicating a silver remedy in the Periodic Table!) and cried easily (*weeping from hopelessness*—if it fits the intrauterine story). He was also a colicky baby from birth on, so we need a colicky remedy! He has difficulty sharing things, even his food, because of *anticipation anxiety* ("I will not have enough"—*anxiety for the future*).

He experienced so much anxiety about whether his mother loved him that he would constantly ask her, "Do you really love me?" His mom's attention was never enough; several times a day he would ask for a hug. He liked constructing things, even building piles with his food. He had great empathy towards handicapped people and fear of accidents (falling into a pit). He feared elevators (falling into an elevator shaft) and sometimes became aggressive when someone invaded his space (*Fear of narrow spaces? Needs an exit?*).

He loved classical music (indicating a silver remedy). All these characteristics must have been present in the expectant mom: Mom's remedy at the time of pregnancy **is his remedy** now.

So I turned my attention to the scene of the possible emotional trauma: an intrauterine event? This was a first child, and he was wanted. Mom experienced lower abdominal pain and thought she might be pregnant but feared at the same time she might have an extra-uterine pregnancy. She went to one hospital where a blood test confirmed the pregnancy but the ultrasound machine was not working, so they rushed her to another hospital with an ambulance (*ailments from: anticipation anxiety; continued excitement; fright*). Then the doctor concluded that this was a normal pregnancy, and that the pain was caused by the stretching of the ligaments surrounding the uterus. The pains persisted and she thought something undetected by the doctors must be wrong (*anxiety, anticipating an event; frightened easily*). She "felt in physical danger" (*fear of death, when alone*). She did not believe the doctor's reassurance (delusions: *is lost beyond all hope to the world; she was about to die; despair in hypochondriasis*). Just at this time, her husband had to travel for an extended period of time. She pleaded with him not to go: "I wanted my husband to stay just in case something happened to me." So she developed fears of *impending disease* (*Argentum nitricum*, 2) and that *something will happen* (*Argentum nitricum*, 2). She also developed the symptoms *desire for company, aversion to be alone* (*Argentum nitricum*, 3) and *fear of being alone*. In spite of her pleading, her husband left since he was reassured by the words of the doctors (causing, in his wife, the delusions: *is despised; is forsaken; repudiated by his relatives; is neglected*). She felt that she could not count on him and told him when he called that he did not need to come back (*childish behavior*). The situation has taken a long time to get over, much longer than the duration of the pregnancy (*hatred, unforgiving to those that have offended; dwells over past disagreeable events; thoughts persistent*). "I called close friends to let them know what was going on with me, just in case I needed their assistance during the night, and I went to sleep worrying" (again, *fear something will happen; forsaken feeling, sense of isolation*). This "what if" emotion was transferred to the fetus, and now we understand this boy.

We see the boy's clinginess and constant need to be reassured of his mother's affection. He asks for hugs all the time, but he has the same feeling his mother had: "Can I trust her when she says she loves me?" The boy also has the same feeling of being despised: "I am dumb, punish me," which may very well feed this delusion. He shows the same anticipation anxiety his mom experienced when she was pregnant. With the boy, this is also expressed in other situations: not being able to share food or toys and fears of narrow places and accidents. The feeling also created anger in the mom, and most anger is based on fear and misunderstanding.

We clearly see several delusions of *Argentum nitricum* in the expectant mother, including delusions *forsaken or deserted* (3), *is despised* (3), *is neglected*, and *is repudiated* (rejection) *by her relatives* and her husband (1). The boy shows this anticipation anxiety in being very protective of his sister, and in his *fear something will happen*, except when he is in a safe environment, surrounded by people he knows (e.g., home, school). He is very protective of his younger sister, just as his mother was toward him while she was pregnant when she would go from one hospital to another to make sure everything was OK. Even afterwards, the mom admits to being overprotective towards him. He needs the "what if/anticipation anxiety" remedy—*Argentum nitricum*!!

Looking at the CD of *Argentum nitricum*, we find the delusions: *he is deserted; he is forsaken and despised*; and *he is lost beyond hope to the world*. Here we see the *Carbon* characteristics of the immature ego creeping in, leading us to understand how the boy's state might be confused with *Pulsatilla*. (*Nitrate* belongs to level two of the Periodic Table, which might also indicate *Nitric acid*). He needs attention and close support. For the mother, support comes from the husband; for the child, support comes from anyone in the home. School is a second home for this child, so he feels protected by the people there and by the building itself. Some *Carbon* selfishness plays a role as well: when expected attention is not forthcoming, he feels neglected. Especially his relatives (or people who play the role of parents/relatives—this may be the homeopath, teacher, guru, etc.) must stand by him at every moment of his life, to shoulder the burdens and deal with the dangers in life: *he looked around as if expecting someone to help him out*, Hering, *Argentum nitricum*. He needs this support to still his anxieties!

A child like this may also be excessively sensitive to a small insignificant snub or offense: *melancholy since an undeserved slight with the fixed idea that he was neglected and despised by his family*—the boy's morbid sensitivity to admonition! Looking again at the mother during her pregnancy, we easily imagine that she suffered from the delusion, *she was about to die* or *she has an incurable disease*. This was transferred to her son, who needs the remedy his mother needed but did not get at that time. Moreover, *Argentum nitricum* is one of the most outspoken remedies for colicky babies! This was often seen when silver nitrate drops were put in eyes of newborns to avoid transference of gonorrhea: Ophthalmia neonatorum. In the past, these "prophylactic" drops brought out the susceptibility to colic in many babies.

Radar software workup for this case:

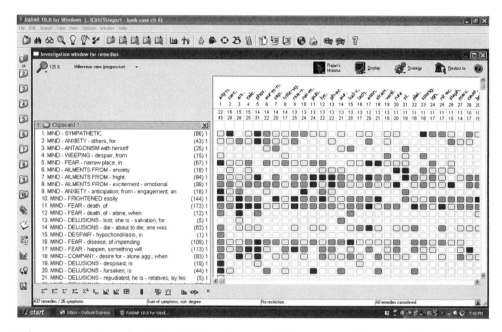

When comparing the CD of *Causticum* and *Argentum nitricum* with each other, the homeopath can see immediately that the CD of *Argentum nitricum, he is despised and forsaken*, fits the patient's case much better than *Causticum's* CD, *about criminals*, which means that crimes are committed all around him, not just to him. It is justice that drives *Causticum* rather than the sense of isolation and forsaken feelings that drive *Argentum nitricum*.

Dream Interpretation

A third method that can be used to uncover the CD is the interpretation of dreams (compensation or parallel dreams). Dreams are not the only content of the unconscious but they are by far the most studied. Fantasies and visions are manifestations of that same unconscious, as they also occur in circumstances of diminished consciousness. This topic will be extensively discussed in my next book, *Beyond Jung: Delusions, Dreams, and Homeopathy*.

How I Determined Criteria for the Core Delusion

Part of the work I have done has been to study extensively the best materia medicas available. My favorites are those written by Constantine Hering, T.F. Allen, Samuel Hahnemann, J.T. Kent, J.H. Clarke, and von Boenninghausen. In my opinion, they are better than any modern materia medicas.

Trying to establish a solid story—a remedy picture based on sound provings, but starting from the CD—I was brought me back to the question: "How do I find the CD of a particular remedy among the manifold proving symptoms as presented in the materia medica and repertory, that is, among the various delusions belonging to that one remedy?" What are the possible criteria for a delusion to be regarded as a **Core Delusion**?

• To me, the first obvious criterion was that among the many different delusions of a remedy, the CD should be either in black type or italics: in other words, this fixed idea is present among most of the provers of this remedy. One example might be the delusion of *Argentum nitricum, he is forsaken and despised,* or of *Aconite, he is about to die.* The latter is a well-known remedy for women in labor with their first child, who may be paralyzed by fear of the impending delivery. Among all its delusions, *Aconite* has only this delusion in bold type. An additional argument to support the choice of *Aconite* as the most typical remedy for this delusion is that *Aconite* is the only bold-type remedy in this rubric and no other remedy has the same intention or meaning as other remedies in this rubric!

• If *all* the delusions of a particular remedy are graded a "1", that is, are listed in plain type, we can try to determine a delusion in which only this remedy is found. For example in the *Silica* proving we find the delusion, *his left half does not belong to his right one,* which expresses the timidity of *Silica* on the outside while he can be a tyrant at home. Only *Silica* is found in the repertory under this rubric. Another example might be the delusion: *he walks on his knees,* which expresses the "smallness" of *Baryta carbonica* on every plane and gives birth to the bashfulness, insecurity, and dependency of this remedy picture. Here, too, in the repertory only *Baryta carbonica* is listed. Yet another example is the *delusion an abyss is behind him,* graded a "2" for *Kali carbonicum,* which refers to the chronic anxiety and threat this remedy picture displays, even while not knowing from what direction the perceived danger comes (the abyss is **behind** her). *Kali carbonicum feels her emotions in the epigastrium* (3) and *has anxiety about the future and her health.*

• Often the essence of the CD is also expressed by other delusions found in the provings of the same remedy. For example, *Lac caninum* has the CD that *he is dirty,* which is also expressed in the delusions, *he is small, she is looked down upon, she is despised, he is short and horrid,* and *he is insulted.* When many delusions express the same theme, this clearly points to the CD. *Kali carbonicum* has the CD that there is an *abyss behind him,* which is also expressed in other delusions of that remedy: *he was about to die; he is sinking; he is sinking in his bed* (reflecting anxiety and loss of control); *he will be murdered,* and *he is sick.*

—

• The CD gives birth to secondary delusions. The CD of *Lachesis* is *he is injured by his surroundings* and *he is wronged*, which leads to further suspicious behavior and secondary delusions such as, *he will be sent to the asylum* and *medicine is poison*. *Aurum* has the CD that *he has neglected his duty and therefore deserves reproach*, which gives birth to secondary delusions: *he is unfit for this world; he has done wrong; he has lost the affection of his friends*; and *everything will fail.*

• Last but not least, a person needing a remedy with one particular CD will always return to his CD after executing a series of defensive compensations and displacements. In other words, the story begins and ends with the CD. No matter how many positive and negative compensations *Aurum* executes, for example, he always will come back to his CD, "I did not do enough, that's why I failed" (*delusion, he neglected his duty*). Or the very psoric *Calcarea carbonica* individual always returns to his CD, *I am about to sink into annihilation.*

• Sometimes remedy provings contain *no delusions* (rarely, but this is, for example, the case for *Natrum sulphuricum*) or there are few delusions and they are also common to many other remedies. The latter example can be found in *Calcarea sulphurica* who, according to the repertory, has only delusions about *seeing visions and ghosts*. In that case, we can get a sense of the "psychic center" or "hidden" CD by examining a strong Aphorism 153 emotion or NWS. In the case of *Calcarea sulphurica*, we see *ailments from anger and vexation*. The significance of this becomes clear when we read a proving for *Calcarea sulphurica* and see the symptom, *lamenting and wailing because he is not appreciated* (Hering). This notion becomes the crux of his fixed idea and all his compensations will originate from this proving symptom. *Calcarea sulphurica shows hatred to persons who do not agree with him* (only remedy in this rubric). So, we could extrapolate that the CD of *Calcarea sulphurica* is *he is not appreciated.*

The *Natrum sulphuricum* picture includes the *Sulphur* element with its need for recognition and a *Natrum* characteristic of being withdrawn and isolated. Here we recognize the dutiful, stoic, realistic person who bears suffering without complaint and without resentment. He is driven by the fixed idea that he needs to take care of people who depend on him. When he fails to do so (e.g., in case of business loss), *he must refrain from injuring himself; fears being left alone lest he should shoot himself*. Again everything (actions, thoughts, and plans) begins with his conviction that his sole purpose is to be objective, factual, and just. In addition, *Natrum sulphuricum* has a strong sense of duty and responsibility (*too much sense of duty*, 2). For him, failure is a dishonor, a poison just as it is for *Aurum*. We should not be surprised then that his hidden delusion may be he *has neglected his duty.*

Do not despair if you can't find the CD. As important as this particular piece of information is, you can still find the remedy by filling in the rest of the pieces. If, at the end of the patient's analysis, a differential diagnosis between two or three remedies becomes necessary, look carefully at the CDs of these remedies and see which ones match the patient picture most closely.

The Patient's Positive Core Delusions

A change of character trait(s), even the acquisition of a delusion, may **appear positive to the patient**. Therefore, as we have mentioned before, do not always expect cooperation from the patient in drawing your attention to what he considers a "good" personal value, one that "serves him well" in life! For instance, professional success may lead to the core *Cuprum* delusion *he is a general*, and *he is an important person*, although it is based on delusions such as *he is selling green vegetables and repairing old chairs*. He may think of himself as a *high commanding officer; a great person*. In other words, the person becomes pompous and arrogant, but sees this as a sign of self-confidence, a useful trait that helps him get ahead in business. But family as well as clients will eventually suffer from his attitude, and (guess what!) so will his business in the end.

How does one acquire a positive delusion? A positive delusion could also be the result of marriage to a successful person. Now the patient can live out his delusion *superior being, not belonging to this world* or *not belonging to his family (Platina)*. Maybe success is achieved in sports or the music world (rock star) and the delusion of being "special" is the result of so-called groupies pursuing him. The "star" does not follow ordinary people's rules, often with the implicit and tacit approval of the public. Even when they are in trouble, for example, they may expect special treatment, as was evident in the trials of Michael Jackson, Martha Stewart, and Kobe Bryant. John McEnroe, the tennis player, used to say to some opponents, "You don't even belong on the same court with me"—not exactly a humble statement. The "star" treatment is not only the province of mega stars. The quarterback of a small college team suffers from the same delusion of superiority as he enjoys his 15 minutes of fame.

The above-mentioned delusions are the most difficult to uncover and to treat because the patient views them as "positive," (he is on the top of the world) so he resists change. Indeed, he sees no reason to change; life is good in the fast lane, at least for him. On the other hand, people around such stars might love to see a change. The patient with such delusions often does not realize that he is living on borrowed time. If the delusional patient's life circumstances change (e.g., the college quarterback does not make it in the pros and becomes a car salesman), he cannot maintain his delusion. His whole world may crumble, often leading rapidly to pathology. So even if he is unaware of it, the patient with a positive delusion is living with a ticking time bomb, which the homeopath would do well to defuse as soon as possible. Simply put, there are **no** positive delusions. Even apparently positive ones can inhibit an individual's maturation process.

Negative Core Delusions

Changes in patients' lives related to sad or **negative** events are more obvious and easier for the homeopath to discover, since they are often the reason for consultation. Someone once said, "Life is 90 percent unhappiness and 10 percent happiness." Obviously, based on that rule, many CDs will find their origin in dreadfully sad events. The "Mind" section of the repertory is full of them. An example might be losing the love of one's life or a soul mate or a very close friend in whom one could confide, any of which might lead to the delusions: *all alone in the world* or *he is friendless* (*Magnesium muriaticum*). Often the negative event is related to situations at work that give rise to feelings of indignation. It may be an unhappy relationship or marriage, leading to the delusions: *cannot succeed in anything* (*Argentum nitricum, Natrum carbonicum*); *being small or dirty* (*Lac caninum*); or *humility and lowness of others, while he is great* (*Platina, Staphysagria*). The event could be related to immigration to a foreign country, leaving friends and family, arriving in a world viewed as full of dangers (*delusion, all alone in the wilderness*) or feeling cut off from all support, undermining one's self-confidence to the point that one now has *Baryta carbonicum's* delusion that *he is walking on his knees*. Or the sufferer might be a teenager or young child trapped in a situation in which the parents take total control (e.g., *Alumina* has the delusions: *he is being beaten; when he says something, it seems to him as though somebody else has said it*). It might be the delusion of someone who is extremely jealous because of heartbreak, leading to the delusion that *he is being sold* (*Hyoscyamus*). These are very negative ideas that may provoke personal pathology, often working as quickly as a silent poison on the mental, emotional, or physical plane, whereas positive delusions do not lead to pathology … as long as the patient can live his "positive" delusion!

An example of the creation of a negative delusion through a horrific event was that of a patient who was raped as a child by her father. When she had metrorrhagia at age 40, she decided immediately on a hysterectomy. She suffered from low energy after the operation. When asked why she "needed" this hysterectomy, rather than resolving the pathology through remedy intervention, she recalled her horrific trauma. It became clear that she had not come to terms with this incident and the shame it brought on her. For her, the place of trauma, the part of her body involved during the trauma, became foreign to her. She behaved as this part did not belong to her, like a cancer, so she didn't hesitate when deciding to remove her uterus—a place of shame. Only a patient who has the syphilitic poison in her (in this case transferred by her father) will resort to such compensation (since it is a mandated hereditary response pattern) to avoid her painful complex!

Negative delusions make up a large portion of such sensitive feeling-toned complexes, but even most "positive" delusions are generated by a painful NWS. Such is the delusion of *Staphysagria*: *humility and lowness of others, while she is great*. For *Staphysagria*, this delusion of grandeur refers to biting your tongue so as not to reveal your deepest emotions (*suffering from pride; ailments from wounded pride;* compare *Palladium, Platina*). These *Staphysagria* emotions, if kept suppressed, must find an outlet on the physical plane as is evidenced in *griping,* **twisting** *pain in the abdomen, colic attacks after indignation, needle-like stitches in the extremities, especially in the muscles* and much later on the emotional plane as we find in the provings, *throwing things around*, in which *Staphysagria* is the only black-type remedy. *She even throws things at persons who offend* (3) but usually in a later stage when the pressure becomes too great or when she is alone at home or in her car. Even *Platina* has these delusions of grandeur (*humility of others while she is great*) generated by her recurrent failures in finding the ideal partner, one she believes to be her sexual and spiritual equal.

Why Resolve and Dissolve a Patient's Delusion?

As long as the patient can and wants to live his delusion, he is most likely not willing to listen, especially if it is a positive fixed idea, as he views it as a good quality! Why should he, since life is dandy for him? The patient will consider the psychoanalyst a madman for daring to put him in such a bad light. "I can't believe he even thinks this of me, where is he coming from?" For example, if the patient knew that the homeopath assigned him the rubric, *contemptuous, hard for subordinates and pleasant and agreeable to superiors or people he has to fear*, the patient might completely disagree with this assessment. This is a patient who is terrified to change because the delusion is markedly fixed in everything he does and thinks. His response is one of resistance and often violence because it is an act of self-preservation. "I never will go to that doctor again," he says, "why pay money to listen to that nonsense." But the homeopath knows that hanging on to this delusion is like dancing on a thin tight rope from which it takes little to fall off!

If it is a *negative* delusion, the patient often feels immobilized and paralyzed as if he is stuck in quick sand. The more he struggles, the deeper he sinks, and no words or encouragement seem to be able to pull him out of it. He needs a way to escape this abyss, and the well-selected remedy is exactly that. His VF, liberated step-by-step from the suffocating feeling of the fixed and torturing CD, in a secondary curative action, "lifts" him out of this deep dark place.

The homeopath can have insights superior to the psychotherapist (not every psychotherapist is Jung), and above all, the homeopath has superior tools at his disposal: remedies. He is able to transform such a person into a patient willing and ready to change. In fact, the remedy has started the transformation already. Because the patient is ready now to understand and look at himself or his shadow side, or in fact to look at the negative influence he has on others, he will not tend to react by running away. Finally, he will become an individual that wants to *be* more, rather than to *have* more, a curse in this present society. By releasing himself from the chains of delusions, he will achieve happiness rather than creating endless anxieties and worries. Indeed, homeopathy will have created an individual that is not focused on the self and alienated from the rest of the world, but a human being with prime concern for and focus on the rest of the world, on his neighbor, whom he will "love as himself." The individual, freed from his CD, is now prepared to be made full and whole again. Anyone whose growth takes this positive direction will also know what is good or bad for him as a *human being*, not good or bad for desired success, wealth, and fame.

"Know thyself" is our goal. It means that man becomes conscious of what is unconscious. This is not an easy process because the unconscious is resistant to becoming conscious. The real process is to gain increasingly more insight into one's self, not just in an intellectual way, but also in an affectionate way. The "heart's" knowledge induces increasing insight in one's secret psyche. The more we succeed in this, the more we are free from all the repressions holding us in captivity. It is just not the knowledge of this, but knowledge combined with the practice of unconditional love and positive insight that propels us towards progress. As the Chinese proverb says, "Reading prescriptions does not make one well."

Does Every Delusion Require a Remedy?

With everything I have told you so far, the answer seems to be yes! But we must never forget what Hahnemann says:

A 252   But if ... one finds in a chronic case that the best chosen homeopathic medicine given in the correct (smallest) dose does not bring about improvement, then it is a *certain* sign that the influence sustaining the disease still persists and that there is something in the patient's way of life or environment which must be eliminated if permanent cure is to be achieved.

One of the most important ways a patient sustains his disease, in addition to the ways discussed in Aphorism 77, is in the way he *thinks*! Our belief system can be very detrimental to our health and growth. This will be slightly influenced by the homeopath's correctly chosen remedy if the disease is created by the way the patient thinks or believes. If the fixed idea or delusion stems from a perverted instinct (miasm), it comes from the VF and the remedy can deal with that. But if the conviction comes from an external source, such as a religion or a tribal custom, then it does not come from a mistunement of the VF. It was the mind and the intellect that created it: from what you see, learn, and are accustomed to (the collective unconsious). This will affect the way patients relate to people and this belief system must be treated by the mind, not a remedy. For instance, Oliver Twist was taught to steal from the rich, which help him survive. And those few pennies stolen would not hurt the person being robbed. This is the "Robin Hood" principle, and it has been transferred by brainwashing techniques used worldwide, even in individual cases like Patricia Hearst who was robbing banks with her terrorist group. Oliver Twist was raised with this conviction, and, rather than a remedy, it is reasoning, by the mind and intellect, that will correct the situation. Hahnemann discusses this concept:

> **A 17** It is possible to create a very grave disease by acting on the vital principle through the power of imagination [and I might add, persuasion] and to cure it in the same way.
>
> A prophetic dream, a superstitious fancy, or the solemn prediction of death on a certain day or at a certain hour have often produced all the worsening symptoms of disease, even to the point of leading one to expect early death—indeed, even to death itself at the predicted hour; this would not be possible without the simultaneous production of an inner change equal to the visible outer one.
>
> By a similar influence, such as an artful pretense or a counter suggestion, it is often possible to banish all the signs announcing early death and to restore health promptly. This would not be possible if this exclusively psychological remedy did not remove the inner and outer disturbances leading to the expectation of death.

In this paragraph Hahnemann stresses the importance of the damaging effects of our belief systems, from religion to personal beliefs. They can all limit us and make us sick; healing can become difficult. A good lifestyle, which requires a balanced upbringing, is very necessary. One can easily see how effective homeopathy **and** psychotherapy work together! *Tolle causam* (remove the cause) is still valuable! If you put a lot of rats in a small cage, they all will get aggressive and neurotic. You give them more space and they calm down: they did not need *Argentum nitricum*!!

Chapter 7: A Remedy Blueprint and Its Core Delusion: The Story of *Lachesis*

Lachesis: An Under-Prescribed Remedy

Lachesis, a polychrest, is one of the most under-prescribed remedies. How can that be? Because *Lachesis* resembles other remedies like *Phosphorus, Sulphur, Staphysagria*, as well as its twin brother, *Lycopodium* (the acute of *Lachesis*). If a patient needing *Lachesis* lacks some the very characteristic physical symptoms of *Lachesis* (e.g., cardiovascular symptoms, throat problems, intolerance to constrictive clothing, and relief of symptoms through discharges), then the homeopath can have difficulty recognizing this remedy on the mental and emotional plane.

LACHESIS PROFILE

Spiritual

P

Strong Ego

Loquacity

Fears

Critical

S

LACHESIS

CD: Recieving an Injury

Killing Rival L

Secondary Delusions

NWS: Grief, Disappointed Love, Jealousy, Fright

Jealousy

Religion-Fanatic

Sex (Sycosis)

Essence and Core Delusion

The essence of *Lachesis* is the caveat or warning about an unlived life or as Edward C. Whitmont called it in his book, *Psyche and Substance*, "the penalty of unlived life" (Whitmont, 1991, p. 151). This should warn us immediately about the possibility of such a situation causing cancer. The *"Carcinosin* state" reflects precisely the same theme: letting others live her life and having no boundaries to prevent this. The appearance of cancer is the final warning to start living your life! In the case of *Lachesis*, we are not surprised to see cancer appearing in the ovaries and sexual organs as they are the center of repressed libido and sexual urges. Besides physical pathology, the penalty of the unlived life is often a series of neurosis, embitterment, and mental decay. With the presence in *Lachesis* of an over-stimulation on every plane, which requires an outlet, we should not be surprised to find **restlessness, anticipation anxiety**, and **hypersensitivity** (*offended easily; sensitive to criticism*) in its primary phase. Often this is followed by **melancholy** and depression. Because *Lachesis* is unable to remove the weeds of egotism and jealousy, he seems unable to cultivate peace in the garden of his heart. Not surprisingly, peace is not manifested externally either.

What is *Lachesis'* core delusion (CD)? She is *about to receive an injury from her surroundings* and *she is being injured and wronged.* As a result, we find suspicion (*full of mistrust*), and the symptom trio (anticipation anxiety, restlessness, and melancholy) mentioned above. Other delusions that express the same thought as the CD include the delusions: *he is persecuted; he is pursued by enemies;* and *he has been poisoned.* The provings state, word for word, *imagines he is followed by enemies who are trying to harm him, and there are robbers in the house and he wants to jump out of the window.* The latter delusions often come after the primary delusion has been allowed to run its course and thus will be part of an advanced mental-emotional pathology, making *Lachesis* one of the most frequently needed remedies for all kinds of schizophrenia.

When it comes to **Carl Jung's consciousness types** (see Chap. 10), *Lachesis* is most frequently the *extraverted, thinking, intuitive* type. According to the circumstances and under the influence of triggers (especially ailments from disappointed love), this extravert can easily become introverted as she can switch from being loquacious to being taciturn. Now we are getting ahead of our story, as *Lachesis* has enough positive tools to try and protect herself, at least initially, from the CD. The question is, are these tools or compensations psoric or mainly sycotic? First, let's answer one question: How did *Lachesis* end up in this "tormented" situation in the first place?

Lachesis and Its "Ailments From"

We have no doubt that *ailments from grief* and *disappointed love* play a big role in the pathology of *Lachesis* (chronic complaints *after long-lasting grief* or *sorrow*). *Lachesis* **IS** a "superior," thinking human being, as are *Aurum*,

Carcinosin, *Sulphur*, *China*, and *Lycopodium*, but of course her reactions to grief are essentially different from those of other remedies. The above-mentioned, "superior" remedies also have a big ego and great ambition, along with plenty of delusions of grandeur, but *Lachesis* is a very passionate person who gets vexed about "competition" with other women, whether in love matters or professionally. This jealousy gets worse on approaching menopause (confirming *Lachesis'* amelioration through discharges). This is a very dangerous time period if the *Lachesis* layer has not been corrected. In Traditional Chinese Medicine (TCM), *Lachesis* belongs to the Fire-Heart element, which cannot live without passion and demands a form of loyalty from her partner that often borders on foolishness. Anger is never far away where grief and disappointed love have occurred. The *Lachesis* woman will find examples among friends who are "spoiled" by their husbands ("he cut my nails for me;" "he always asks, can I do something else for you?", etc.), and she will use those as markers to determine how much she is loved and cared for by her own husband (**delusions of reference** according to Jung[1]).

We see the intensity of *Lachesis* on the emotional plane: there is no middle ground, only the high road, like an Olympic flame that burns with desire forever! Indeed, the flames of this fire need very little impetus to get out of control and, driven by *foolish* and *irresistible jealousy*, they can lead to hysteria, compulsion, and to all kinds of unexpected, impetuous actions which, in her mind, are totally justified. *Lachesis* is often an example of a person who is partially overcome by her unconscious. The condition at first can be temporary when it is a matter of emotional upset. But in a state of violent emotion (foolish jealousy), she says or does things out of proportion, which she regrets afterwards when reason is somewhat restored. Even the most normal individual is not immune to this danger, but *Lachesis* can bring this outburst to unsuspected heights. And not much is needed: disappointed love, grief, jealousy, or hatred for her rivals is often strong enough to reverse the relation between the ego losing control and the unconscious temporarily gaining the upper hand. *Lachesis* is a "well-spoken" lawyer at heart: you cannot win an argument with a *Lachesis*! To everyone else, she is as suffocating as a boa constrictor and appears utterly ridiculous since her jealousy often has no real basis, except in her imagination.

---

[1] Both *Hyoscyamus* and *Lachesis*, two of the most jealous characters, have many delusions of reference. Jealousy is a great cause of delusions for these two remedies. When they are driven by it, any small circumstance, gesture, or word can produce the grossest misjudgment. Under suitable conditions, these characters will "jump out of their skin" and temporarily imitate the insane. Often, *Lachesis* or *Hyoscyamus* will jump to the conclusion, during their first moment of anger, that they have been deliberately injured or insulted (delusions: *has suffered wrong; is injured by his environment*). The danger, of course, is that *Hyoscyamus* and *Lachesis* may cross the line from neurosis to psychosis. The homeopathic history contains many cases of frank insanity that required one of these two remedies.

A perfect example of such foolish jealousy is as follows:

> I am constantly accusing my boyfriend of looking at other women and thinking of other women while we make love. Recently, I gave my boyfriend a gift certificate for a massage, but I wanted to be in the room, watching everything that happened. When I found out we could not be in the same room, I cancelled the appointment. After hearing him complain about his bad back, I rescheduled the massage. Then after the massage, I yelled at him for having some other woman's hands all over him. I am thinking of leaving him because he has been "tainted" by someone else (this example came from *The New Mexican, Annie's Mailbox*, August 30, 2005).

Of course, the newspaper columnist suggested that this person seek counseling. Indeed, allopathy does not have one single drug to allay jealousy whereas homeopathy has at least 50!

Lachesis' Compensations

How does a person compensate for all the events (*grief, disappointed love, anger, and horrible things affect her greatly*) that can lead to the CD of *Lachesis? Lachesis* possesses a *strong ego*, which helps explain the patient's reactions and compensations, as well as the origin of the CD. In haughtiness and pride, she is not far behind *Platina* and *Lycopodium*, the most outspokenly arrogant people. Interestingly, *Lachesis* shares the Never Well Since (NWS) triggers of *Platina* and *Lycopodium*: vexation, mortification, and disappointment. However, these remedies have a much different reaction to this assault on their ego. *Platina*, depending in what stage she is in, eventually chooses one of her extreme outlets (e.g., sex, religion) and pursues her path in that way. *Lycopodium* often maintains his quest for power, attempting to remain at the top of the social ladder through defiance, cynicism, hard work (*delusion, neglects his duty*), and false arrogance as he exhibits an almost dictatorial behavior (*dictatorial, speaks with a voice of command*) with *want of amativeness* in men (3). *Lachesis* and *Lycopodium* are both "thinking" remedies, but *Lachesis* typically belongs more to women. *Lachesis* wants to be successful, above all, in relationships; success in her career comes next. *Lycopodium*, more often used for men, sees a successful career as being the most important thing, as do *Nux vomica* and *Sulphur. Lachesis* places the greatest importance on her career only by default (i.e., when she is frustrated sexually and her husband cannot match her intensity of possessive love). So for *Lachesis* it is more a perception than a reality that she is not loved, and her jealousy makes her incapable of maintaining her mask in the relationship.

Thus, the delusions of these remedies will take different forms. *Lachesis*, belonging to the Fire element, is prone to more hysterical "heart-love" delusions, expressions of the strong anima, the snake being a symbol of the human anima (e.g., delusions: *she is beautiful*; *she is going to have a heart attack*). *Lycopodium*, belonging to the Wood-Liver element, will have more delusions about his place in society, his image, and his success at work—the animus or sword at work (e.g., delusions: *he neglected his duty*; *he is presumptuous*; *he is unfortunate*; and the CD: *everything will vanish*).

MALE CD VERSUS FEMALE CD

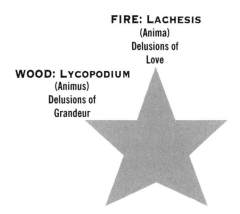

FIRE: LACHESIS
(Anima)
Delusions of
Love

WOOD: LYCOPODIUM
(Animus)
Delusions of
Grandeur

Platina and *Lycopodium* end up being queen and "false" guru respectively (a real guru serves people, does not insist on being served by others). *Lachesis* is a tormented soul in the sense that she does not understand why her often foolish and out-of-control passion is not returned with an equal show of "love." *Lachesis* and *Platina* are both "spiritual" remedies and thus act and talk as though they were under superhuman control. *Platina* is a little harder, even a little more crude in her actions, than *Lachesis*, who is much more easily influenced by "being mesmerized": *thinks she is somebody else and in the hands of a stronger power; she acts like she is charmed and she cannot break the spell.* Thus, *Lachesis* will more likely be part of a cult or group rather than a leader like *Lycopodium* and *Platina*.

To bolster her ego, *Lachesis* possesses something else that makes her superior to *Platina* and *Lycopodium*: her **loquacity**! *Lycopodium* speaks in a more dictatorial way towards his inferiors (even *abusive and insulting towards subordinates*; often with *anger from contradiction*). This brings to mind *Nux vomica*, who like *Lycopodium, employs every possible means for his ambition* (also *Platina*!). At the same time, *Lycopodium* speaks differently in the presence of his boss: *he is a flatterer* because he knows he needs to be on good terms with his boss in order to reach that coveted position of power. *Platina* can be loquacious, abusive, and insulting, especially a child toward her parents (*Lycopodium*). She can be a *braggart* and a *boaster*, and squanders her money through ostentation

(*Veratrum album*). This is part of *Platina's* "beauty," which takes the form of an ice maiden rather than a warm, sympathetic person. In her deeper pathology (luetic phase), *Platina desires to be silent* and is *indisposed to talk*.

Lachesis speaks in different ways depending on her state of pathology. When in balance, *Lachesis* is a witty and brilliant conversationalist. She has *quick comprehension* and *mental activity with almost prophetic perception*. *Lachesis* stops you in the middle of your sentence as she knows the rest already, even worse for you, she knows the question before you have asked it. With *Lachesis*, the *ideas are abundant and no sooner does one idea occur than a number of others follow in quick succession*. She is active, lively, and vivacious. Usually her speech reflects all this: *wants to talk all of the time; inclination to be communicative; vivid imagination and extremely impatient at tedious and dry things* (she doesn't like small talk!). She has the most *extraordinary loquacity, making speeches in very select phrases, but jumping off to the most heterogeneous subjects. One word leads into the midst of another story. This exceptional loquacity is marked by a rapid change of subject; she jumps abruptly from one idea to another* (whereas *Platina* has a *wandering speech; repeats the same things*). *Lachesis talks, sings, or whistles constantly*. True to her snake nature, her tongue will be used to hurt in a very refined but cynical and critical way. *Lachesis* hurts with a word while having a smile on her face. For *Lachesis*, talking is the therapy that soothes her CD.

This loquacity is of an imminently sycotic nature, indicating clearly to the homeopath that *Lachesis* is a very sycotic remedy, rather than a psoric one—very different from *Calcarea carbonica*, a strong psoric remedy, someone who likes to ramble about all the little things he suffers from, but never speaks eloquently. (If he ever waxes loquacious, *Calcarea carbonica* always wants to mull things over before he becomes a nuisance by talking about his little issues and ailments.) Any compensation of *Lachesis* will be an exaggerated one with an intensity to it that matches the remedy's sanguine nature. At least initially, for the more stable *Lachesis*, the loquacity is an outlet of a rather positive nature that can serve them well—a good lawyer, politician, teacher, or preacher!

"Loquacity" also appears in letters or emails! If you, as a homeopath, always get a lengthy answer to your follow-up questions, all about "small" complaints but very detailed and always urgent, pleading, and self-absorbed, you can call that loquacity! Their messages are blow by blow accounts hurled at the homeopath, which makes you think of an *Arsenicum* personality who is consumed by anticipation anxiety and restlessness! An out-of-balance *Lachesis* really suffers from the delusion, *she is doomed*, and in her panic, reason goes quickly out the door.

How else can *Lachesis* get away from her CD? In accordance with her haughty and proud character (*Lachesis* is graded a 2; *Lycopodium* and *Platina* are graded a

), *Lachesis* believes she is in contact with powerful people (*delusion, is under powerful influence*). Furthermore, she may be of the opinion that she has a special relationship with God: religion becomes another outlet for this tormented soul. She seeks safety by communicating with people in high positions (e.g., writing letters to the President of the United States). This is similar to *Veratrum album* who thinks he should be received by the most famous people in order to advance his own social status. As usual, we often see a religious compensation when the sexual outlet is either suppressed or impossible, for example in puberty (*Kali bromatum, Platina, Lilium tigrinum, Lycopodium, Veratrum album*).

Lachesis' religious compensation also matches the intensity of the sexual outlet and is equally of sycotic (exaggerated) nature (religious monomania and even fear of being damned). Often the female teenager will invoke religious compensation when sexuality awakens, if she has been brought up in a strict religious milieu where the topic of sex is taboo. They might go into the streets to preach to people about the end of the world (*Veratrum album*). Male teenagers are more likely to engage in thrill-seeking and dangerous behavior. As usual, the extreme can turn into its opposite: we can find rabid atheists among *Lachesis* people (i.e., *Lachesis* patients are fanatical). *Lachesis* always has this compelling quality to their beliefs: they are totally convinced and reject any dissenting opinions.

A "positive" compensation for *Lachesis* is the **sexual outlet**. If the sexual outlet is available, that is, not suppressed by family mores (there is a big difference between growing up in a 1960s pot-smoking environment and a strict religious family!), it also takes an extreme form. The **male** either becomes a Don Juan (*great excitement of sexual desire*) or more commonly is so fixated on his partner that he becomes as demanding sexually as a *Lycopodium* male, easily transforming his wife into a *Staphysagria* or *Sepia* state. This quickly leads to a negative cycle: *foolish jealousy* transforms this passionate person into a man who normally is in firm command of all his actions, but now loses it at the slightest emotional event. This is a perfect example of the "thinking" *Lachesis* getting into trouble when the inferior, more primitive "feeling" side becomes dominant. This superior, thinking individual is now confronted with situations he cannot handle, and it manifests itself in very foolish behavior and all kinds of jealous reactions: *jealousy with rage; jealousy with saying and doing things he normally would not do;* and *gentle husband becoming brutal from jealousy.* To dull those very painful feelings, *Lachesis*, once on this negative pathway, does not shy away from alcohol, which he can tolerate very well (even a *debauched life*) and which fuels his jealousy and suspicion even more. We must not forget that *Lachesis* is **THE** remedy for hereditary familial alcoholism!

The **female** *Lachesis* may look for love in all the wrong places (like *Platina*), while taking it one step further. She does not hesitate to become a prostitute with the naïve conviction (remember the "feeling function" **IS** primitive) that she will find love and romance in this environment. As the *Lachesis* state worsens from the cessation of menstrual flow or excretions (e.g., during menopause, which often in her mind signals the end of her femininity), the sense of having to compete with younger women can erupt into the open with the force of a volcano. If there is a younger rival, thoughts of killing that person surface and even murder is not uncommon!

Turning to the Negative Pathway

The negative pathway leads immediately to **fears** (a negative sycotic reaction), which are a direct consequence of the CD and which fuel the CD immensely. Besides the *fear of being damned* and believing themselves to be doomed and unable to escape their fate, they have immense fear of *robbers*, of *water*, and of *going to sleep* (since this always aggravates their condition). He *fears he will die during his sleep* from a heart attack; *anxiety about the heart.* The *Lachesis* patient seldom experiences *refreshing sleep as their sleep [is] restless with many dreams and frequent waking and dozing again.* Another component to their fear of sleep is that during sleep, the unconscious escapes any control mechanism and can exact its compensatory revenge in dreams. Other *Lachesis* fears are of *people walking behind her,* of *snakes,* of *suffocation* (turtlenecks are not tolerated); *fear of narrow places, elevators, swimming under water,* but especially fear of *an incurable disease* such as cancer; *fear of the cholera; cramps in calves from fear with nausea,* and *heavy feeling in the abdomen.* In her paranoid, fragile state, but long before she truly "loses it," *Lachesis* starts fearing that she is *becoming insane.*

Lachesis is a major remedy for cardiovascular diseases (strokes and heart attacks). She often *experiences constrictive pain, oppressive chest pain and palpitations with numbness in arm, improved by sitting up.* Often, during fits of jealousy, heart symptoms and fainting will occur: *after a jealous (hysterical) quarrel, she put both hands on her chest and cried out, "Oh my heart!", then fell down and was in an [asphyxiated] state for 24 hours; no pulse could be felt, breathing hardly perceptible.* If she is not sleepless from fear of heart attack, *she is sleepless after domestic calamity* (relationship problems), *woken up by terrible dreams.*

As we proceed further into the negative cycle, jealousy becomes ubiquitous. Jealousy (combining egotism, lack of true love, and an expression of possessive love and suspicion) will affect the "thinking" function of the *Lachesis* person as her inferior "feeling" function now becomes the dominant function. The superior, thinking person has become an inferior, feeling person. Where before she was witty with a great memory, now *her mind is confusing and wandering; there is even great dullness of mind with bodily weakness. She is even tempted to commit suicide* as secondary delusions take hold of her spirit. Everyone around her becomes suspect. *Hyoscyamus* has the delusion that *he is going to be sold,* and that *a lover is hiding behind the stove. Lachesis* also feels that she is going to be replaced by someone else, someone younger and more beautiful, of course. Even kind gestures appear to her as threats. Her husband wants to give her a remedy for those pulsating headaches but this leads immediately to the delusions: the *medicine is poison* (*Hyoscyamus*) and *he is about to be poisoned.* And if her husband does not poison her, *he is probably scheming of sending her off to the asylum* (*delusion, asylum, insane, sent to*). At this point, it is not difficult to see that *Lachesis* has come full circle and returns to her CD.

We can see that the *Lachesis* person is at a great risk of crossing the line from neurosis (hysteria) to psychosis and schizophrenia (*has two wills*) whenever additional problems arise. This leaves *Lachesis* in a state where she cannot cope with reality any more. The normal balancing act of the conscious and unconscious is interrupted; dangerous, uncontrolled elements of the unconscious, unexpected manifestations from this darkness, crash into the conscious and overwhelm the ego. Schizophrenia is the result! In this real psychosis, the unconscious elements could not be assimilated by consciousness. Whoever is attacked by such fantasies and visions is either seized by an immense fear that he is going crazy or he thinks he is a genius. I have seen both. But whatever road the patient was forced on to, he is at once isolated from others, who are unable to understand him. Formerly unconscious contents are rising to the level of consciousness and disrupt the hegemony of the ego. It is here that the homeopath can shine. Such patients need understanding, sympathy, and the certainty that they can share their crazy ideas with someone. This relieves them of the fear of falling into the dark gaping abyss. The homeopath does not close his books when the patient says, "I am seeing ghosts" or "I am conversing with God." He will say: "Describe these visions and conversations for me." These symptoms are some of the most peculiar Aphorism 153 symptoms.

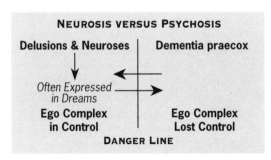

NEUROSIS VERSUS PSYCHOSIS

Delusions & Neuroses	**Dementia praecox**
Often Expressed in Dreams	
Ego Complex in Control	**Ego Complex Lost Control**

DANGER LINE

Lachesis: Example from Jung's Clinic

I have plenty of *Lachesis* cases from my practice, but I believe it would be interesting to look at a case of schizophrenia from Jung's early years (1906). What is especially interesting about this case is that, from early on, *Lachesis* was indicated. However, in spite of Jung's best efforts over many years, the only result was the manifestation of secondary delusions belonging to *Lachesis*. In fact, the patient seems to cover almost all of *Lachesis'* delusions. What would have been the outcome if Jung had been a homeopath? It is also a great example for today, because such a patient would either be put on a strong anti-psychotic like haloperidol or locked up in a modern asylum.

I have inserted rubrics (in italic type) into Jung's text as it appears in *The Psychogenesis of Mental Disease*. These rubrics **all** belong to *Lachesis*, so we're confident that it is the simillimum! This case also reminds me of a time when, as a young medical student, I was confronted with a similar case: a schizophrenic young man who would come to me with tears in his eyes, showing me the newspaper where a murder was described and of which he accused himself. I wish I could see him now! Following is Jung's case.

This is the story of a dressmaker, unmarried, born 1845. The patient was admitted in 1887 and since then has remained permanently in the asylum. She has a severe hereditary taint [not explained by Jung; probably luetic miasm]. Before admission, she had for several years heard voices [*delusion, hearing voices*] that slandered her. For a time she contemplated suicide by drowning [*suicidal disposition by drowning = Lachesis*]. She explained the voices as invisible telephones. They called out to her that she was a woman of doubtful character, that her child had been found in a toilet, that she had stolen a pair of scissors in order to poke out the child's eyes [*delusion, had committed a crime*]. (According to the anamnesis the patient had in fact led a thoroughly respectable and quiet life.) [Only *Lachesis* is found in the rubric *delusion, voices, hearing-confess things she never did.*]

Now and then the dressmaker used peculiar expressions and in general spoke in a somewhat pretentious manner [*speech, bombast; speech, extravagant*]. The patient produced vivid delusional ideas [*ideas abundant, clear*]: she had a fortune of millions; at night her bed was stuck full of needles [*delusion, injured by her surroundings*]. In 1888 her speech became more and more incoherent [*speech incoherent; Lachesis* is graded a 3!], and her delusions unintelligible: for instance "she owned the monopoly" and "legions perish of death by suffocation." In 1890-91 the delusions became more absurd: "she became Queen of the Orphans" and "proprietress of the Asylum" [*haughty; egotism*]. 1895: patient felt paralyzed and claimed she had consumption [*delusion, doomed, being; and feigning to be sick*]. 1896: I am Noah's Ark, Empress Alexander, Mary Stuart [*delusions: is a great person; of errors of personal identity; she is someone else; and insanity, loquacious; megalomania*]. 1899: patient tormented at night by thousands of snakes.

At present the patient is, as ever, a diligent worker [*industrious; Lachesis* is graded a 2]. When she is not actually talking of her delusions to her doctor, her behavior and speech are quite orderly, though there is an unmistakable affectation such as is often found in elderly spinsters who try to create a substitute for unsatisfied sexuality by the greatest possible perfection of demeanor [outlet for *Lachesis: loquacity for suppressed sexual desire*]. There is no imbecility. Her speech is only altered where her delusions are concerned: otherwise she speaks normally, reports on what she has read, and defines ideas in a clear way [*abundance of ideas, clearness of mind*], provided they do not touch the complex.

During tests and analyses she shows great readiness to cooperate and takes visible pains to make herself as intelligible as possible [*haughtiness*]. She is always calm and there is nothing striking in her outward behavior. She is always pressing for interviews, hoping finally to convince us and thus reach the goal of her desires. While at work she whispers her "power-words" to herself, stereotyped sentences or fragments of sentences with a very strange content [*speech, repeats same things; loquacity, busy; loquacity in selected expressions*] ... Remarkable is that she brings out her strange delusions with marked lack of affect [*indifference, apathy*].

The psychic activity of the patient is completely taken up by the complex: she is under the sway of the complex; she speaks, acts, and dreams nothing but what the complex suggests to her [*dream, as if in a*]. In normal people and hysterics, we find striking or linguistically odd reactions, always at the critical places, and especially words from a foreign language [*speaks in a foreign tongue*]. These correspond here to neologisms, which the patient describes as "power-words". [In order to understand these power-words, Jung asked the patient to form associations to these words—that is, he would say the word, and the patient would add other words.] For instance, responding to the power-word Socrates, she said: 'pupil-books-wisdom-modesty-his teachings-falsely accused-I was the best dressmaker-fine professorship *delusion, of fancy illusions; haughtiness*]—prison-slandered by wicked men-brutality.' These associations did not come smoothly but were constantly inhibited by 'thought-deprivation' [*vanishing of thoughts while speaking; Lachesis* is graded a 2], which the patient described as an invisible force that always took away just what she wanted to say [*delusion, is under a powerful influence*].

In her delusions she says, 'I am like Socrates, and I suffer like him' [*delusion, she is someone else*]. With a certain poetic license, she says, 'I am Socrates' [*delusions: identity, errors of personal identity; is a great person*]. Here is a clear instance of deficient discrimination between two ideas: every normally functioning person can distinguish between an assumed role or metaphorical name and his real personality [*delusion, wills, two*]. Changes in speech normally occur very slowly but in this patient the changes take place rapidly [*loquacity, changing quickly from one subject to another*]. Responding to the stereotyped word 'silver,' she associates: 'I have established the mightiest silver island in the world,' and 'highest eloquence' [*loquacity, in selected phrases; speech, bombast, worthless*] and 'speech is silver, silence is golden,' among others. Silver is also speech; hence she possesses the highest eloquence. She has dreams of men coming into her room at night armed with daggers, swords, lances, or revolvers: invariably sexual symbols, the wounding weapon being a symbol for the penis [*dreams: amorous; lascivious*] (Jung, 1989, pp. 99-101).

Jung's conclusion concerning this case is that the patient, brought up in miserable circumstances and poverty, is creating in her psychosis a complicated and senseless fantasy-structure (i.e., the patient describes for us, in her symptoms, the hopes and disappointments of her life, just as would a poet). The poet speaks the language of the normal mind, therefore most normal people understand him. However, the patient speaks as if in a dream (*dream, as if in a*). When Jung told her impatiently to speak louder, she answered irritably, too. At this moment, the "telephone" called out: "Now they are getting in each other's hair!" In all these conversations the "telephone" has the character of an ironically commenting spectator, a split-off personality (*wills, two*). Can the homeopath have any doubt about his prescription in this case?

Note: In my next textbook for the professional homeopath, *Beyond Jung: Dreams, Delusions, and Homeopathy*, I hope to provide approximately 100 remedy blueprints, similar to this one for *Lachesis*.

Chapter 8: The Patient's Constitution

Question 9: Who Is the Patient? What Is His Temperament, Constitution, Attitude, and Dominant Function of Consciousness?

Mandatory Response Pattern

In normal circumstances, a constitution is preset at birth. It is a combination of the parents' constitutions. If the mother experiences abnormal circumstances while pregnant, the expected constitution may be mistuned by that event. For instance, a child is born *Natrum muriaticum* because of a mother's grief while carrying the baby; or it comes into this world needing *Tarentula* because the mother experienced ailments from unrequited love. In cases of in-vitro fertilization, the baby may be affected, since the mother often experiences anticipation anxiety, fear, discontentment, etc., while she is waiting to know the outcome of the procedure; even after she knows she is pregnant, she may be fearful of losing the baby.

In my opinion, according to the teachings of Carl Jung and homeopathic philosophy, constitution is **the inherent tendency to respond automatically along certain qualitatively predetermined, individual, characteristic, and fixed response patterns**. Constitutions can be described by characterizing these fixed response patterns. Any attempt to stop the response pattern typical of a certain constitution and to enforce a pattern that is different from the inborn automatic one, always meets with fundamental resistance; in the long run it proves impossible! That is to say, our reactions to events are *compulsive, not elective*. Each individual reacts according to an innate predetermined emotional pattern that makes it impossible for him to respond otherwise.

Many psychotherapists claim that man is by no means a product of heredity and environment but ultimately decides for himself. The eminent Dr. Viktor Frankl[1] for one, speaking of his period in concentration camps, claims that in spite of social restriction, people reacted differently: some were hopeless from the beginning and committed suicide; others were heroic in their suffering, always giving

---

[1]Victor E. Frankl, MD, PhD (1905-1997) was the author of 32 books, professor of neurology and psychiatry at the University of Vienna Medical School, and founder of Logotherapy and Existential Analysis. During World War II, he spent three years in concentration camps.

hope and even sharing their sparse food supplies. Dr. Frankl claims they all still had the freedom of choice in how to respond, but I disagree with this: the predominant miasmatic state (see Chap. 12) together with the constitution, more than environment or decision-making fueled by the right education, will dictate the outcome for each individual. Without a doubt, those who opted for suicide were acting out of their inherited syphilitic miasm, while those who helped out others were strongly psoric in nature, a true gift from their ancestors.

For example, someone who is constitutionally choleric cannot respond in a phlegmatic way to criticism, even if he tries hard to do so. His attempt will only lead to a partial, artificial, and unconvincing reaction. In the same vein, we speak of psoric-allergic constitutions, or of *Sulphur* or *Nux vomica* constitutions, etc. This also means that the simillimum cannot change the vitriolic, violent response pattern of a *Nitric acid* personality (*delusion, he is engaged in lawsuits*) into a placid, yielding *Pulsatilla*. Pathology and suffering can only be overcome by adapting oneself to one's constitution, by trying to manifest its positive rather than its negative side, that is, by smoothing out the rough edges and polishing the diamond within us with the help of the simillimum or through long-term psychotherapy and analysis. And guess which one I would choose!!

The Value of the Constitution in Determining the Simillimum

The constitution is the foundation that will determine much of your fate. A *Phosphorus*, a *Carbon*, a *Kali*, a *Magnesium*, or a *Sulphur* person will react differently to the same hardship. *Sulphur* and *Magnesium carbonicum* have the tools for surviving hardships: tenacity, cunning, intelligence, street smarts, drive, and perseverance. A Carbon person or a *Phosphorus*, with either an undeveloped ego or a lack of boundaries (*likes to be magnetized*), might be utterly depressed and succumb when faced with a similar event. The question therefore arises: is the constitutional temperament a valid factor to consider in finding the simillimum?

Kent wrote a short lecture titled, *Classification of Constitutions Useless in Prescribing*. In that lecture, Kent opined:

> Why should we attempt to classify constitutions as an aid in prescribing? It is a fatal error to classify constitutions, as no two are sufficiently similar, when observed by a genuine homeopath to form even a common class. The physician who prescribes on a diagnosis is a failure, except for his chance shots. The symptoms that represent the morbid constitution or disorder of the individual are the ones that the skillful prescriber always seeks. Symptoms that are uncommon in one constitution are common in another, because such uncommon symptoms are common to some diseases and uncommon to others (1994, p. 272).

Indeed, we can all recognize that each human being is a constellation of characteristics that serve to distinguish him from others, characteristics such as body build, color of hair and eyes, etc. that are **within the health of the person** and cannot be altered by homeopathic remedies.

But we must **contradict** this idea immediately as Hippocratic constitutional temperaments do not only deal with characteristics that are within the state of health. This system includes the Yin and the Yang, positive and negative characteristics, as well as the symptomatology that these body/mind types suffer from when under the stress of specific disease triggers. This typology, developed by the ancients, was intended to determine the effects of triggers in order to understand susceptibility, dyscrasia, and predisposition of individuals—just as Hahnemann expresses in Aphorism 73 regarding **occasional sporadic diseases**. The word "temperament" has different levels of meaning. In general, it means state of mind and disposition. In particular, it means the physical and mental organization of the body. Specifically, it refers to the Hippocratic constitutional temperaments (choleric, sanguine, phlegmatic, and nervous). Disease is a mistunement ("Verstimmung") of the vital force (VF) and the temperament.

Hahnemann writes about *Pulsatilla* in his *Materia Medica Pura*:

> Hence the medicinal employment of *Pulsatilla* will be all the more efficacious when, in affections for which this plant is suitable in respect to the corporeal symptoms, there is at the same time in the patient a timid, lachrymose disposition, with a tendency to inward grief and silent peevishness, or at all events a mild and yielding disposition, especially when the patient in his normal state of health was good tempered and mild (or even frivolous and good-humored). It is therefore especially adapted for slow, phlegmatic temperaments; on the other hand, it is but little suitable for persons who form their resolutions with rapidity, and are quick in their movements, even though they may appear to be good tempered (1989, p. 345).

We see that the terms "constitution" and "temperament" were used in homeopathy from the beginning. Indications of this phlegmatic "earth type" are followed here by Hahnemann's counter-indications: rapid decisions and quick movements, traits belonging more to a sanguine-fire type like *Phosphorus*.

Another **very** important facet is the change in disposition and temperament that may occur during an acute disease. This absolutely must be investigated as it plays an important role in finding the acute remedy. The more drastic the change, the more important it is. When using the von Boenninghausen method, the mental/emotional symptoms are taken into account only at the end of the investigation in order to differentiate between close remedies.

Hahnemann stresses the importance of emotional changes in acute diseases:

A 213 Therefore one will never cure according to nature—that is, homeopathically—unless one considers the mental and emotional changes along with the other symptoms in all cases of disease, even acute ones, and unless for treatment one chooses from among the remedies a disease agent that can produce an emotional or mental state *of its own* similar to that of the disease as well as other symptoms similar to those of the disease.

Thus *Aconitum napellus* will seldom or *never* cure either quickly or permanently if the disposition is calm and undisturbed; nor will *Nux vomica* if it is mild or phlegmatic; nor will *Pulsatilla* if it is glad, cheerful, and willful; nor will *Ignatia* if it is steady and without fearfulness or irritability.

Hahnemann makes it clear that a perfect prescription follows Aphorism 7 (totality of the symptoms) and states:

A 5 In addition, it will help the physician to bring about a cure if he can determine the most probable *exciting cause* ... In this he should consider: the evident physical constitution of the patient (especially in chronic affections), his affective and intellectual character, his activities, his way of life, his habits, his social position, his family relationships, his age, his sexual life, etc.

Aphorism 5 reflects the mind/body complex of a human being. What do they do? How do they live? What characterizes their sexual behavior, their intellect, etc.? These are all constitutional factors that must be taken into account when selecting the perfect prescription.

In Constantine Hering's extensive provings published in *The Guiding Symptoms of Our Materia Medica*, he paid special attention to the corresponding Hippocratic temperaments. About *Pulsatilla* he wrote:

Persons of indecisive, slow, phlegmatic temperament; sandy hair, blue eyes, pale face, easily moved to laughter or fears; affectionate, mild, gentle, timid, yielding disposition. Especially suitable for good-natured, timid people, inclined to grief and submissiveness. Women inclined to be fleshy. Delicate features, color of face readily changing (1997, p. 650).

Hering's examples in *Guiding Symptoms of Our Materia Medica* are very useful as they show us physical constitutions during the state of health and how the medicinal diseases induced by the remedies (provings) transform them. If it was observed that specific remedies brought out more symptoms in one type of constitution than another, these statistics were recorded. Homeopathic remedy provings led to well-known characteristic symptoms. For example, *Nux vomica* is described as being well adapted to irritable, thin, dry, bilious, and choleric temperaments, whereas, *Ignatia* is suited to women of hysterical, changeable, and nervous temperaments. According to Hering's provings, *Phosphorus* is well adapted to tall slender persons of sanguine temperament, fair skin, delicate eyelashes, fine blond or red hair, with quick perceptions and a very sensitive nature. *Arsenicum* is well adapted to the over-anxious, chilly, and nervous temperament. In the materia medica of Hering's *Guiding Symptoms*, he describes *Stages of Life and Constitution* for each remedy, indicating that such and such remedy fits and acts well on a particular constitution and temperament. Note that he is not saying that the remedy causes such constitutions!

By adding the other concomitant symptoms of the patient, we may conclude that this slow, weeping, warm, and gentle temperament is manifesting *Morbus Phlegmatica Pulsatilla*, while the fat, chilly, morose temperament is manifesting *Morbus Phlegmaticus Graphites*. They will always be phlegmatic temperaments, but they may need several different remedies in their life to reach optimum health. **The individual has a phlegmatic temperament, not a remedy.** A remedy is what they need based on their exhibiting symptoms. Hippocratic constitutions are helpful in selecting homeopathic remedies, as their character-istics are part of the overall totality of the symptoms. Our bodies manifest symptoms as a guide or directive to put the homeopath on the right course; and we can only manifest those symptoms that express our innate constitution. Thus Kent shows little understanding of the Hippocratic system, thinking it is only about the *unchangeable* characteristics of individuals in the state of health.

Baron von Boenninghausen, in his *Lesser Writings*, supported Hahnemann's view: "A contribution to the judgment concerning the characteristic value of symptoms" (1991, p. 105). During the great homeopathic congress held in Brussels, Belgium, von Boenninghausen proposed a prize-question concerning the value of symptoms. Since no one came up with a suitable answer, it was von Boenninghausen himself, who had come to homeopathy from the practice of law, who answered the question in the form of the ancient lawyer's hexameter of which the first question is: *Quis?* Who? Who is the individual who suffers? In this question, von Boenninghausen states:

> ... must stand at the head of the image of the disease. To this belong first of all the sex and the age; then the bodily constitution and the *temperament* (emphasis added); both if possible, separated, according to his sick and his well days, i.e., in so far as an appreciable difference has appeared in them ... The spiritual and dispositional individuality of the patient here gives the most important, often almost the only deciding points.

—

Thus, von Boenninghausen taught us that it is important to understand the natural predispositions of the constitution in the state of health in order to perceive that which is strange, rare, and peculiar in the "dis-eased" state of that same individual. All innate temperaments and their mixtures have both positive and negative states as well as their own symptomatology. Homeopathic *Pulsatilla* can, for instance, enhance the positive traits of a phlegmatic personality while the negative ones diminish or disappear all together: slow, perspiring, morose, and anxious phlegmatics (negative traits) can change into active, happy, and outgoing phlegmatics, ready to contribute to society (positive traits).

Nobody ever claimed that a person would become taller or their hair color would change under the action of a remedy, but these traits have nothing to do with the degree of suffering. The fact that Hering mentioned blue eyes and sandy hair in his provings doesn't mean that *Pulsatilla* will create these features. I have treated plenty of patients needing *Pulsatilla* who didn't have blue eyes or sandy hair! In those same provings, however, Hering did mention "slow phlegmatic" temperaments because he found that *Pulsatilla* had little effects on sanguine and choleric temperaments.

What is therefore important to the homeopath is to pay attention to a *change* in temperament in an individual, pointing to the development of a disease (acute or chronic), a change that will aid us in selecting a remedy.

By now, it should be abundantly clear that the constitution is one of the grand sum of triggers in humans that predisposes them to certain chronic miasmatic conditions and that homeopaths must take all these triggers into account in their prescriptions if they want to select the true simillimum. Hahnemann was the first physician of his time to integrate constitutional factors such as inherited constitutions as well as spiritual and emotional temperament, miasms, and predispositions thus advancing the work of Hippocrates regarding constitutions and temperament.

A Question Regarding Constitution and Provings

Here is a question posed by one of my excellent students: "My understanding of provings is that they are conducted on the healthy. In Hering's *Guiding Symptoms* there is a section called, *Stages of Life and Constitution*. Many of the people mentioned in this section are not healthy but suffer from many illnesses listed. Can someone explain this to me?"

Dr. Luc's answer: "Indeed, Hering stressed differentiating between 'cured symptoms' (the ones from clinical cases) and 'proving symptoms.' Like

Hahnemann, Hering said, 'The homeopath must make such discriminations, and those clinically confirmed symptoms are less important. But one must mention the difference between these symptoms otherwise perplexity instead of lucidness would be developed through the combination. It should be considered as a matter of the highest importance, never to mix indiscriminately, symptoms *reported as cured* (*not* having been observed on the healthy), with the symptoms produced by the drug'" (Hering, 1997, pp. 12-13).

In the aforementioned *Stages of Life and Constitution*, Hering discusses not only the different stages of life (from newborn to old age and anything in between), he also mentions cured symptoms, which as stated above, are of less value (graded a 1) than proving symptoms. Most of this refers to Aphorism 5 of the *Organon* in which Hahnemann mentions: "... the evident physical constitution of the patient ..., his affective and intellectual character, his activities, his way of life, his habits, his social position, his family relationships, his age, his sexual life, etc." Moreover, in this section of Hering's *Guiding Symptoms*, the homeopath can often find a temperament suited to a particular remedy. Or the homeopath can find information regarding the kind of patient for which the remedy is suited based on the patient's sensitivity, disposition, or appearance (thin, obese, scruffy, etc.). Hering also mentions other characteristics that people may having including: lax fibers and muscles; awkward gait; indolent behavior; or lack of reaction, etc.).

Some other examples of the stages of life and constitution include: ill-natured children; children who are excitable; nervous persons; bilious temperament; lean persons; old people and children; hypochondriacs; fat and sluggish with body parts fat and legs thin (*Ammonium muriaticum!*); weakly hysterical woman; a strong, well-developed man of phlegmatic temperament; stout women who lead a sedentary life; scrofulous children, etc.

Extraverts and Introverts

Before Carl Jung arrived at his "four functions of conscious," he introduced a classification of his patients based on two other types: *extravert* or *introvert*. Each of the four function types can be further broken down as one of those two. Jung postulated that individuals adopt differing habitual attitudes toward life, which determines their interpretation of experience. In other words, these are psychological modes of adaptation. The **extravert** defines himself in terms of his relationship with the events in the surrounding world, while the **introvert** sees the world in terms of his own situation within it. According to Jung and to more modern psychotherapists, these attitude types are neither a matter of conscious choice nor of inheritance. While I agree with the first part of the statement, I respectfully disagree with the second part. The dominant active miasmatic state is indeed predetermined and is not a conscious choice (see Chap. 12), but the attitude type will certainly be influenced by the presenting, predominant miasmatic state.

For example, the syphilitic and the mixed cancer miasms are introverted, as a rule, while the sycotic and the mixed tubercular miasms are extraverts. The psoric person who is looking for support can be both an introvert, because he mulls things over and theorizes about everything, and an extravert, because he looks for support from others and enjoys the company of family and friends. That's why two children from the same family can be of opposite types! Just as the patient may progress through different miasmatic stages, either because of homeopathic treatment or through lack thereof, they can change their attitude type throughout life. For example, a sycotic, extraverted teenager can turn into a depressive introvert later in life when the syphilitic miasm has replaced the sycotic one as the dominant miasm.

Weaknesses and Strengths of the Attitude Types

The two attitude types are more easily recognized in our patients than the four functional types, which we will discuss later.

• The extravert has a tendency to want to be noticed (e.g., *Argentum nitricum*, *Argentum metallicum*, *Palladium*, *Platina*, *Lachesis*, and *Sulphur* in their initial phases), that is to say, he is always "on the offensive," projecting his image and attempting to be a leader.

• The introvert, on the other hand, wants nothing better than to disappear and remain incognito. He is always slightly on the defensive, guarding his privacy fiercely. He is the silent leader, bringing up the rear; the one someone can fall back on, feeling secure in his arms.

• The extravert wants to join the action and get on with whatever they're doing without delay (*Tarentula, Phosphorus, Sulphur, Lachesis, Nux vomica,* etc.)—often impulsively. But he is confident and takes full advantage of opportunities by easily adapting himself to different situations.

• The introvert observes, hesitates, and mulls the situation over, making him slow to act (e.g., *Calcarea carbonica*).

• The extravert (often a sycotic thrill seeker) is attracted and fascinated by new, unknown situations to which he adapts easily.

• The introvert has a cautious psoric approach to unknown situations. He organizes his life in advance and does not like to improvise.

• The extravert (e.g., *Argentum nitricum, Ignatia,* and *Pulsatilla,* all graded a 3 for impulsiveness!) acts first and thinks later. He decides quickly and acts with vigor and immediacy, just the opposite of the introvert.

• The extravert enjoys the noise and bustle of the city, crowded shopping malls or souks in the Middle East.

• The introvert looks for refuge in his quiet home, away from the city center. The more crowded the place, the more he is reluctant to visit it.

• The extravert longs for the good opinion of others (*Palladium*) and is influenced by public opinion and the majority views.

• The introvert looks within for self assessment and is rarely convinced by the opinion of outward sources.

• The extravert wants to influence others through his words (e.g., loquacity: *Lachesis, Sulphur, Phosphorus, Lycopodium*) and possesses natural authority and a commanding temperament.

• The introvert influences others inadvertently through his silent deeds (e.g., *Aurum, Natrum sulphuricum*). (The loquacious person is often the "blabber"—the tactless gossip. Most people avoid telling anything to an the extravert if they don't want their personal issue broadcast everywhere by the next day.)

• The extravert projects and exaggerates his moral values so he does not have to recognize his corresponding vices. (There is nothing high that does not come from lowly roots, or as Nietzsche put it, "The tree whose branches reach to Heaven has its roots in Hell.")

While the extravert cultivates many friendships, often not carefully selected (e.g., *Phosphorus* who is seeking to connect to the rest of the world and is driven by her core delusion (CD): *all alone on an island*), the introvert approaches friendship as something sacred, a gift, deserved by few (*Natrum muriaticum* in its third stage; *Sepia*). The extravert hates to be alone because he is then forced to see himself (introspection), something he does not feel comfortable with. The approach and investigation of the unconscious arouses panic and fear in the extravert. Secrets simply don't exist with extraverts. Their motto: "If no news is available, send rumors." They carry their "hearts on their sleeves," and often get burned by sharing their feelings. Introverts don't tell secrets; privacy should be maintained at all cost. Of course, extraverts are secretive about *certain* aspects of their lives, a strong sycotic trait. This is not contradictory to the notion that the sycotic miasm is mainly an extravert in its expressions. The secret part is often hidden by other exaggerated and extraverted expressions. Take for example the charismatic preacher who hides his secret sexual life; examples of this type have become public often in the last decades.

The extravert avoids anything that would dull his optimistic and creative outlook. Whatever he does is done with enthusiasm, warmth, and the total conviction of impending success: "Life is beautiful!" His excessive optimism often borders on careless confidence in unknown situations and lacks investigation of the true possibilities. The word failure is not in his vocabulary and risk-taking is part of business as usual (*Nux vomica*). He likes to embellish reality and is rarely objective. Of course, he can quickly get bored if positive results are not forthcoming and will change his profession, or his major at the university, or even his spouse. Often he undertakes too many things at the same time and runs the risk of not finishing any of them. Success may be obtained through unbridled enthusiasm or through ruthless behavior; he may display choleric or sanguine temperament, foul language, or push himself to the point of ruining his health.

The introvert is more cautious, anxious, and maybe timid, with a phlegmatic or nervous temperament. He sees obstacles even where none exist (e.g., *Silica, Gelsemium, Lycopodium*, and *Aurum* who *sees obstacles everywhere occasioned by fate and then by himself*) and is guarded about the future and any task at hand. Failure is definitely an option and a real possibility. This can lead to irresolution and missed chances as the extreme introvert may lead a life of inertia, even suffering from a lack of lust for life. In the end, he may be more efficacious because he acts according to a successfully proven formula, using objectivity as a guideline, analyzing everything without passion. He can count on others since he is a rather silent but trustworthy leader, one who leads through deeds rather than extravagant speeches. Unlike the extravert, he desires to reach the highest distinction in his assigned role and is willing to put in the time it takes. He is also successful because of what he demands from others, and of what he demands from himself.

To the extravert, introspection (i.e., fishing around in his unconscious) is full of danger, and he does everything to avoid doing it. For him there is definitely only one world: the one he lives now, conscious reality as he sees it. For him, dreams are only dreams, annoying little stories that are waved away the moment he wakes up. He finds enough confirmation and reassurance in the outside world that "all is well and all will stay well." He may be hooked on books with titles like "How to Get Rich in a Year!" He may not hesitate to approach or even transgress the line of criminality to secure success.

The introvert, on the other hand, cultivates his interior world and often keeps an intimate journal. He relies on his introspection to derive satisfaction, comfort, and the confidence to face everyday events. Dreams are of great interest to him and he loves to analyze their meaning. His unconscious world looms as big as his conscious world, and he derives great satisfaction from cultivating his shadow side. Failure to do so would only increase the ever lurking presence of anxiety. Books with a title like "Psychology of the Unconscious" are a guide for him, and justice and honesty are likely to be primordial in his life. He compensates for his vulnerability through his lucidity.

The extravert is the social butterfly, the life of the party, mixing effortlessly with everyone, lighting up the room through their presence or their firm command of any interesting topic (e.g., *Phosphorus, Medorrhinum, Lachesis, Lycopodium, Sulphur,* and *China*). Friends fill his appointment book. He is easily mesmerized by his friends, and he can just as easily mesmerize others. Charisma, flirtation, and communication are his tools. People cannot help but notice the big brash extravert with the booming laugh, often to the point that later on, they are unable to recall anyone else, as if the extravert had used up all the oxygen in that room. The female extravert's bright slash of lipstick and provocative clothes (giving expression to her art of seduction) often denote a sexual prowess used to conquer others. Much of the true extravert's time is spent in sensual pleasures, outings, games, card playing, receptions, films, etc. The introvert would look-

—

down with disdain on such superficiality. The introvert approaches any individual more cautiously; few gain his trust or overcome the elaborate defense mechanisms he has built up. The introvert is not a good mixer, she is the wall flower. She barricades herself against others' influence and has few close friends. Only kindred spirits are allowed into her sanctuary.

The extravert is forgiving, possessing an air of superiority and confidence mixed with delusions of grandeur (delusions: *he is a great person; he is a general; he is a prince*) and has no difficulty enjoying others' successes. The introvert may become envious and very critical, finding a hair in every bowl of soup, calling the extravert a superficial gad-about while she herself is driven by lack of confidence, feelings of inferiority, and mistrust. Her delusions are often linked to affairs of the heart or religion (delusions: *wretched when looking in the mirror; is persecuted; all alone in the world; is in contact with a higher being or God*, etc.).

Calling the introvert a "stick-in-the mud," the extravert can make a fool out of himself, be the butt of jokes, and probably look on it all as a positive experience, whereas the introvert surrounds himself with barbed wire and hockey gear in order to avoid any embarrassment. The introvert's frugality, pedantry, and cautiousness clash with the extravert's boundless generosity, camaraderie, and impulsivity.

The Neuroses of These Two Attitude Types

The most frequent neurosis of the extravert is *hysteria*, belonging to the Fire Element in Traditional Chinese Medicine (TCM). This is a sycotic, exaggerated response to the immediate environment: a constant tendency to make himself interesting and noticeable may include the realm of fantasy, which often includes behaviors such as, lying, boasting, and exaggerating the facts. If the extravert also possesses an exaggerated conscious attitude, his unconscious attitude will be infantile and archaic, possibly leading to a nervous breakdown or to abuse of drugs, or infantile egotism. Of course, mental/emotional extraversion will lead to the typical extravert's exaggerated and theatrical physical symptoms as perceived in *Ignatia*: "globus hystericus," sighing, trembling, sobbing, convulsions after grief or admonition ... all are sycotic expressions.

The introvert, belonging more to the Water Element in TCM, is more likely to be overwhelmed by *anxieties and phobias*, which lead to indecisiveness and awkward behavior, isolating that person even more. But guess who's in control? As much as the extravert thinks **he** is, he's no match for the introvert: water conquers fire!

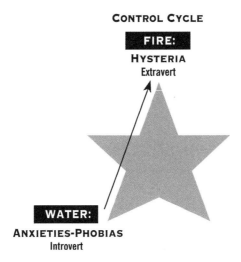

CONTROL CYCLE

FIRE:

HYSTERIA

Extravert

WATER:

ANXIETIES-PHOBIAS

Introvert

At first glance, it looks like the introvert is a social loss, a misfit. In his search for quietude, he is easily accused of being aloof, cold, arrogant, distant, anti-social, proud, obstinate, egotistical, and cranky. But we must not forget that for each individual there exists an objective and a subjective world, just as the wholeness of man is made up of a luminous conscious world and a dark unconscious one. Turning towards the subjective has just as much value as paying attention to the objective. For these two types, there is just a difference in priorities; in each individual, there is a predominance of one of the two sides. However, both types would do well to avoid any one-sidedness. To be a more complete person, it is better to exercise both attitudes.

What is of value to the introvert may be of no value or interest to the extravert. My wife (an introverted, intuitive *Carcinosin*) went on a day trip with an extravert friend who declined to visit museums and wanted to go shopping. This didn't meet with much enthusiasm from my wife, but as they went from one shop to another, they hit on one where old medical instruments and books were displayed. This delighted my introvert wife who all of a sudden appeared to be the extravert as she talked animatedly to the shopkeeper about the history of these treasures. Meanwhile, the spirits of the extravert friend fell, and she could not wait to leave, because she was now becoming bored and withdrawn. In other words, that particular shop produced a role reversal: my wife became the extravert, her friend the introvert!

Marriage and the Attitude Types

The previous anecdote brings us to the topic of marriage and relationships. We know very well the old adage "opposites attract," and indeed, it appears that an ideal marriage would consist of the symbiosis of these two opposite people, the introvert and the extravert, each unconsciously complementary to the other. While one partner reflects and investigates, the other takes the initiative and acts upon the reflection of his partner. A life full of roses and no thorns? Alas, we know such roses do not exist. When the extravert man reaches the point in life where he has been successful in his career and has reached his goal (i.e., a comfortable retirement), he now has time to occupy himself with his introvert partner and starts meddling in her business. He does not realize that until that point, both have been standing back to back, each looking at their own horizon and guarding it zealously. Now suddenly, they are facing each other and may discover that they have never known each other. "For better or for worse, but not for lunch, my dear!"

Here, the conflict between the two attitude types is almost unavoidable if each wants to impose their attitude on the other. (The exception, of course, is the happy, "ideal" person who will be able to recognize and appreciate the other person's value. Unfortunately, such people are rare.) We must remember that the extravert does possess an introvert attitude, which has remained dormant, undeveloped, and more or less unconscious (most extraverts rarely exercise their introvert attitude). And of course, the opposite is true for the introvert.

At the moment of retirement, he faces the world with this undeveloped weak side, and it is a daunting task. Only those who have inner courage and have come a long way on their path of individuation are successful in applying the "weak side" for the benefit of the marriage. For the others, the end of their "ideal" symbiosis will come in the form of a rude awakening, causing untold difficulties between the partners. Accepting the value of their partner is tantamount to reducing their own value, except of course for those few "normal" or should we say, exceptional people who have exercised both attitudes. Indeed, throughout their lives, the introvert and the extravert have often cultivated opposite interests (just as they have lived separate lives). Now, when both partners no longer have to face external necessities, like making a living, the symbiosis that is hanging by a thread may shatter. We can see why the typical *Aurum* personality (having occupied a high position as a CEO, a powerful physician, lawyer, or a high-ranking military man, etc.), when he retires, may fall into a great depression. He is not able to face his unconscious life and the life that was "unconscious" with his partner. He feels lost; life has ceased to have any importance (delusion, *he is unfit for this world*). Boredom, anxiety, irritability, succumbing to a heart attack, and even suicide are common consequences.

Attitude Types: Fixed or Flexible?

A change in the attitude type **is** possible either through psychoanalysis (which might take a long time) or through the homeopathic simillimum. These attitudes may also *spontaneously* alternate, often linked to certain periods in life, for example, living with a different culture. Different countries have different attitudes, often influenced by a mild or a severe climate. The Italians, in general, are more extraverted (i.e., have a sunnier disposition) than the Nordic peoples of Finland and Lapland, where darkness and bitter cold rule for six months a year. The Renaissance period was one of extraversion versus the more introverted Middle Ages.

Family circumstances, such as early responsibility or ailments from domination, can change the extraverted *Phosphorus* into an introverted *Sepia* or *Carcinosin* type. Under such circumstances, this individual is forced to adapt by assuming an unnatural attitude, violating his innate disposition. This can lead to neuroses as well as to physical ailments, especially auto-immune disorders and cancer! Clearly, puberty, which awakens the miasms (especially the sycotic miasm, linked to the awakening of sexual hormones), is a period of extraversion whereas menopause, with a decline of estrogen, is more of a Yin (introverted) period. Other hormonal changes—during menses, pregnancy—can lead to such a switch from extravert to introvert. A perfect example is *Lachesis*, who, being a very passionate person, normally has most of his compensations in an outspoken extraverted attitude: loquacity; rambling; jumping from one topic to another; jealousy; and increased sexual behavior. During pregnancy, *Lachesis* tends to resemble *Natrum muriaticum*, as she may become withdrawn, averse to company, and feel sadness, especially on waking. Another example is the remedy *Aristolochia clematitis*, who also goes from extreme introversion to extraversion: happy one moment and crying the next. They are extraverts mainly during menses, but otherwise are predominantly introverts (with a sense of solitude). This is expressed in changing attitudes towards food—going from bulimia (the extravert) to anorexia (the introvert).

Even the different stages in our remedies, especially when linked to the miasms, will show that over the evolution of the remedy type, the person can go from extravert to introvert. *Natrum muriaticum* is a perfect example. During the first, psoric phase, a very naïve and impulsive *Natrum muriaticum* certainly portrays an extravert-feeling type as evidenced by the provings: *laughs and sings all day long; she laughs immoderately; she is amorous, amative; lascivious and exposing herself.* But already during the middle phase (sycosis with its exaggerated efforts to stay in a relationship) and even more in the final (isolated) syphilitic phase of withdrawal,

—

refuge, loneliness, and hatred, the extravert-feeling type develops an introvert-feeling attitude. Proving symptoms that demonstrate these changes include: delusions, *talks with the dead, sees visions of the dead, is wretched when looking in the mirror; company, avoids company and enjoys thinking about past sad occurrences although it exhausts her*, etc.

—

Chapter 10: The Four Functions of Consciousness

Hippocratic Temperaments and the Functions of Consciousness

In Carl Jung's *Analytical Psychology: Its Theory and Practice*, (Jung, Lecture One, 1968, pp. 16-20), he discusses four different functions that can be distinguished in each individual's consciousne . He uses the categories *sensation, thinking, feeling,* and *intuition.* He explicitly says that he does not use this terminology in order to put his patients into a box or a category, but he finds it valuable for himself to have terminology when dealing with and describing people of different make-ups. I think an analogy can be made to the four Hippocratic temperaments (choleric, sanguine, phlegmatic, and nervous) that may help homeopaths analyze a patient's state and progress.

Together with the predominant miasmatic state and the inherent constitution, we can use the observations of Jung and Hippocrates when predicting the pathway (positive or negative) a patient will take, propelled by their core emotion. An individual cannot be choleric and phlegmatic at the same time, since these are opposite states. If a patient is characterized as being choleric, it goes without saying that the term phlegmatic is excluded.

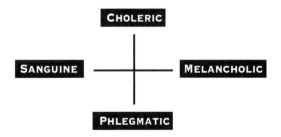

An individual characterized as yielding and torpid would have nothing in common with an angry individual; these two feeling states are at opposite ends of the scale. The nervous-melancholic type belongs to a side of the spectrum that is diametrically opposite to the sanguine personality. The melancholic type (Water element in Traditional Chinese Medicine [TCM]) and the sanguine type (Fire element in TCM) are opposites in the same way. The more fiery the individual is, the less melancholic; the more hysteria, the less depression, and vice versa.

—

On the other hand, an individual can be choleric as a primary temperament and have as a secondary or auxiliary temperament either sanguine or melancholic, which will then modify to some extent the dominant temperament. The choleric-sanguine person will certainly react like a fiery volcano, while the choleric-melancholic type will be prone to alternations between anger and sadness. These alternating states are well known in homeopathic remedy provings.

Clinical Use for Homeopaths

Homeopaths can use classification into the various temperaments and constitutions as a valuable tool. Such classifications are not only useful as an aid to understanding patients (and prescribing for them according to Aphorism 281), but are also a particularly helpful instrument when the homeopath is called upon to explain children to their parents or husbands to their wives (or vice versa). They are also helpful in understanding interpersonal difficulties that arise between people.

Jung viewed his typology in exactly the same way. It is interesting that Jung resorts to a classification similar to that proposed by Hippocrates. Why only *four* functions? The number four has been regarded from time immemorial as a sacred number and a symbol of wholeness. We find the mystic four, the essence of all existing things, the basic number in, for example, the four arms of the cross or the four sections of a mandala.[1] The four different functions square off in pairs and are diametrically opposed to each other (Jung, 1968, p. 17).

On the one hand, we have thinking and feeling functions, which are rational functions. Both of these necessitate judgment and evaluation, whereas sensation and intuition are the irrational types. In the latter two functions, everything is based not on reasoned judgment or interpretation, but upon the absolute intensity of mere perception. That does not mean that the latter two types are "unreasonable or illogical." The functions of judgment *are* present but largely in an unconscious or latent way, so that sensation and intuitive types can be called highly empirical. Thinking can also be identified with the head, intuition with the sympathetic nervous system, feeling with the heart, and sensation with the limbs.

---

[1] "Mandala," a Sanskrit word, means circle. Its symbolism embraces all concentrically arranged figures, all circular or square circumferences having a center, and all radial or spherical arrangements. The drawing of a spellbinding circle is ancient magic. Whoever is within this circle has security and safety. It is a place of protection, a holy and inviolable retreat. A circle or globe, roundness of an object, and a mandala also express perfection, completeness, and totality.

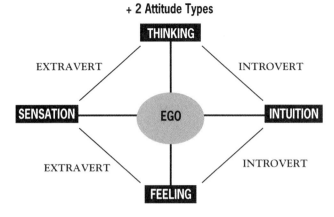

JUNG'S 4 FUNCTIONS OF CONSCIOUSNESS

+ 2 Attitude Types

Each of the two non-diametrically opposed functions has a secondary importance: they have an *auxiliary* or *complementary* function that will change the nature of the person, and each is useful only in so far as it serves the dominant function without claiming superiority. In other words, this secondary function has a different nature from, but is *not antagonistic* to, the primary or superior function. If we think of the functions of consciousness as arranged in a circle, then the most differentiated function is generally the carrier of the ego and is usually coupled with an auxiliary function. The so-called inferior function, on the other hand, is unconscious and for that reason projected upon a non-ego. For instance, the thinking type can have either sensation or intuition as a secondary or auxiliary function. Each of us can work with the secondary auxiliary function to make us more balanced A person's dominant function is already maximally differentiated. A third function is rarely available to the average person because it is in the shadow (we can also call it latent) but it can become accessible to a person depending on their degree of health. The fourth archaic and primitive function is, as a rule, entirely beyond the control of a person's will. So an individual can be a thinking-sensation type but rarely will he be a feeling type at the same time! Further differentiating and elaborating the auxiliary functions (in this case feeling and intuition) will take the edge off the superior function and create a more balanced person! But for the thinking type, feeling will always remain his Achilles tendon!

Two of these functions, the most differentiated one (thinking in this example) and its auxiliary function (sensation), are conscious and therefore masculine. In dreams they are pictured, for instance, as father and son. The unconscious functions—the primitive function and the other auxiliary function, intuition— are, on the other hand, seen as mother and daughter respectively. Since the contrast between the two auxiliary functions (sensation and intuition in this example) is not nearly as great as the contrast between the differentiated and primitive function, it is possible to raise a third rather unconscious auxiliary function to the level of consciousness and thus become even more masculine. The exercising of three possible functions of consciousness is part of the process of individuation.

The fourth and undifferentiated function of consciousness (feeling, in our example) is **an integral part of the unconscious** and when it is made conscious, it will bring along with it the dark contents of the unconscious. This represents a battle between opposites (thinking-feeling) and the thinking individual, who views himself as a very reasonable person, would desperately attempt to keep himself from falling under the spell of what he deems, "murderous nonsense and absurd superstitions." But if the fourth function is forced out by some event, it will possess this reasonable person, until, as he says, "I finally came to my senses after that small incident when I didn't feel quite like myself."

PRIMARY FUNCTION OF CONSCIOUSNESS & SUBORDINATES

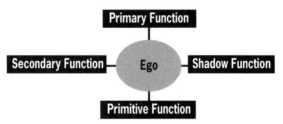

Exterior factors (emotional events especially), miasmatic influences, and innate constitutions will determine the predominance of one of the four basic functions, leading the individual to the function that will undergo the most pronounced development (the dominant function). This dominant function gives the conscious attitude its direction and quality. Just as the homeopath recognizes "combination" constitutions (noting that one function will always be predominant), Jung also allows in practice the appearance of combination function types, individuals who combine practical intellect with sensation (*Lycopodium*), artistic intuition with feeling (*Phosphorus* and *China*), and philosophical intuition with vigorous intellect (*Sulphur*). As we can see, the secondary function, the unconscious auxiliary function, tempers and supports the conscious primary function, as long as it does not try to take the leading role. It can never be a function whose nature is opposed to the leading one, however.

Feeling can never serve as a secondary function to thinking, for instance, since it is the diametric opposite of the thinking function. The only time thinking and feeling functions can be closely associated is among children and primitive peoples (the primitive mentality).

The undifferentiated and inferior function (or fourth function) in a person is always his Achilles heel, an open door through which anyone can enter. It is a Trojan horse, attacking him at those unfortunate moments when circumstances force him to operate temporarily in his fourth function mode. No wonder the thinking type guards his feelings like a jealous lover. While the reaction of his superior function surfaces quickly and can therefore always be counted on, his "fourth function" is so primitive that it takes extra effort to dig it out of the mud, so to speak. The fourth function is relentless, however. Neurotic symptoms, dreams, and other manifestations of the unconscious, such as mildly uncontrollable and "incomprehensible" moods, as well as strong emotional reactions of any kind (from falling in love to blind rage) are often expressions of that inferior side trying to assert itself and a proof that this inferior function has been activated.

While most people will not be very clear about the function type to which they belong, homeopaths can use this system of categorization as an additional tool. Over and above determining the temperament and constitution, determining the function type can help homeopaths better understand their patients and lead to a better prescription. Armed with this knowledge, the homeopath will be able to avoid serious blunders in dealing with patients, especially when it comes to communication. Let's see how the homeopath can increase his successful intervention with his patient through the intelligent application of Jung's types.

Applying the Four Functions When Communicating with Patients

Different homeopaths have different ways of introducing themselves and the theory of homeopathy to their patients. These practitioners all mean well and are often convinced that their method is the best.

One of my students said to me, "I always give patients a 15-minute explanation before I start the first consultation: I explain what the principles of homeopathy are, what to expect, how homeopathy works, etc." I could see that he was convinced that this was the right way to start a consultation and that every patient would be grateful for having such an understanding healer. But is this really true for every patient one sees in the office? The homeopath might be surprised to learn that what one patient appreciates, others would be offended by.

In the past, I made the mistake of sending a lengthy questionnaire to each patient before the initial consultation. Much later I realized that rarely did I get the information. I really wanted. Even before I discovered Jung, I quickly learned that "going with the flow," adjusting myself to each patient individually while conversing in the consultation room, worked much better. In a sense, I was lucky as this came naturally and instinctively to me. Jung's typology made it all very clear, however. I think studying Jung's version of types is very practical for every homeopath and healer.

Recognizing the type of patient you have in front of you is a great advantage for the homeopath. In order to get the message to the patient and thus increase the likelihood of therapeutic success, the homeopath has to communicate to people in their superior function. Without that, no contact is established. The "thinker-homeopath" cannot talk exclusively intellectual jargon to his "feeling-type" patient (e.g., explaining homeopathy in terms of quantum energy to a *Phosphorus* patient). He might as well talk to a wall. The patient will feel utterly lost, even insulted, the homeopath will be frustrated, and no bond will be established between them. The "feeling-homeopath," on the other hand, will upset the thinking, "hurried" patient (e.g., *Sulphuric acid, Nux vomica*), who wants rapid practical solutions to his problems. Too many questions about his feelings (although information concerning them is very necessary) will turn that patient away from this "new-age nonsense!" The newest rage among some homeopaths is to ask the patient continuously about his "true feeling" (although they incorrectly call it "sensation"). "But what do you *really* **feel**?" is their mantra, since they want to capture the essential, core feeling. The thinking person will view this homeopath as a freak, and the feeling person will keep him busy with garrulous and useless jargon.

How to proceed then if the homeopath wants to discover the emotions of the thinking type? It will be necessary to trick these "intellectual" types (who, by the way, often suffer from delusions of grandeur) by asking them innocent questions about their plans, performances, friends, etc. and also by dropping names of famous people (to whom they relate easily). The homeopath will need to mention how he himself has had fears or anxieties about certain events. I never hesitate to express my own fear of heights, as that can help the patient feel more comfortable and more willing to reveal a weakness. At this point, it should be clear why "fixed" introductions about homeopathy are a hit or miss tactic, depending on the type of patient you have sitting in front of you. The truly blessed homeopath has the gift of leaving his own dominant attitude type behind and engaging the patient in **his** superior function.

You Are What You Are: Accept, Cultivate, and Cherish It!

While everyone might think he belongs to the superior function type (delusions of grandeur!), it is imperative to accept in advance that none of these four types is superior to another, nor is one of the two dominant attitude types more desirable than the other. They each make their own contribution to this world.

In order to establish the actual order of the four function types in your own case, you must possess strict psychological self-criticism, something that is not given to everyone. Whatever dominant type you are, it is the one best suited to you and how you compensate and adapt to the world around you. Adaptation to the environment naturally always occurs via the superior function. This is again analogous to the homeopathic constitution: if you are a *Phosphorus*, this means you will adapt according to a predetermined, compulsive response pattern, which will be different from that of a *Sulphur*, for example. The *Sulphur* pattern is not preferable to that of *Phosphorus*: you are what you are!

Unfortunately, circumstances arise in which the individual is forced to adapt via his inferior function, rather than his natural superior one. This will always lead to unhappiness, neurosis, and maladjustment. Consider for example the countless *Phosphorus* or *China* artists, who were forced by rigid, thinking parents to "study something decent," to become a lawyer or doctor, something that "earns money." The child is thus forced by his parents and the pressures of education to rely on an undifferentiated and undeveloped inferior function. This constitutes unhappiness: such persons always feel lost, inadequate, and unnatural about their actions and thought processes. This mechanistic behavior is a betrayal of their natural superior function, which has been suppressed by the rigid standards of parents and society. The consequences of a total imbalance between superior and inferior function can be devastating: one side of the diametrically opposite pairs is almost emptied or suppressed when it happens forcefully, as in the case above. The inferior function is pushed to perform and as a result, this pair of opposites can disintegrate, leading to neuroses, even to a total dissociation or splitting of the personality as in schizophrenia!

I remember such a case: a fragile, thinking person was so pushed by her mother to become a world class pianist that she totally dissociated at age 17, never to leave the mental institution where she still lives today at the age of 70. Energy lost by her consciousness passed into the unconscious and activated its contents: repressive feelings, painful complexes that then overflowed and invaded her consciousness with such brutality that it split her mind.

THE BIRTH OF PSYCHOSIS

CONSCIOUS LIFE   UNCONSCIOUS LIFE

Sometimes it is not a person that forces a change in function. It can be a *situation* that demands that the person handle the event with his inferior side. For example, a feeling type who usually seeks to fulfill the demands of reality by means of empathy may easily encounter a situation that can only be solved by thinking. In this case, the feeling function might break down and the progression of the psychic energy or libido ceases. This stoppage of progression of libido can easily lead to the birth of neuroses or psychosis, as we have seen above. Indeed, when the dominant function is operating in an individual confronted with a situation, there is a state of regular interaction and mutual influence between the pairs of opposites, allowing a successful adaptation and a balanced progression of the psychological processes. This stoppage of the libido is always marked by the breaking up of the pairs of opposites, however. The longer this stoppage lasts, the more the value of the opposite function increases. Instead of a mutually balancing cooperation, the pairs of opposites attempt to suppress each other, leading to conflict and, in the case of a successful suppression of one of the opposing forces or functions, a splitting of the personality ensues. More often, this first sets the stage for the birth of a neurosis. Take the *China* personality, for example. It is the disunion between the thinking and feeling functions that will lead to its well-known persecution paranoia (delusions: *he is persecuted; he is hindered at work*).

Try to Be Complete, Not Perfect

Could the individual increase the efficacy of these four functions through *education* so that they become equally differentiated? For example, "I am an individual who has 25 percent of each of these functions?" That would surely make a perfect human being but per definition this is not possible. Perfection can never be reached, as echoed by a life-long homeopathic treatment of the individual, who needs constant adaptation and readjustment to the many different complexes and triggers in his life. Perfection would make dreams obsolete, since compensation for this perfect conscious life would not be necessary; the link with the unconsciousness would thus be lost. What a boring world it would be if everyone was perfect; it's the difference in people that gives spice to our existence!

I think perfection (an impossible goal) is not to be strived for; trying to be "complete" is a better purpose. "Complete" refers in homeopathy to the reduction of the negative or syphilitic side, or rather the subduing of a patient's active miasmatic state(s). "Complete" refers also to balancing the Yin and Yang in TCM and to an investigation of Jung's "shadow-side." "Complete" is accepting what you cannot change. Try rather to diminish the negative or Yin aspect of your constitution and temperament while increasing the Yang or positive side. Our goal of achieving psychological totality, individuation, is met when we have made three of the four functions and both attitude types as conscious and available as possible.

Trying to be more complete also means that you fulfill something you are able to achieve rather than running after something that is hopelessly beyond your reach as an individual (a pipe dream). Often, I daydream about being an opera singer, and that it would increase my anima if I could be Maria Callas, but I know the shower is the only place where Dr. Luc is allowed to sing. So it will not be for this life, and I had better dedicate my time to something I **can** achieve.

Being more complete also means that the individual should behave in the same way whatever the circumstances. Most people adjust their attitude in public, thus dissociating into two people: one in the outside world (a mask) and one in "inner" or private life (reflecting the soul). It is easily observed here that a "splitting" of personalities is something that can happen in perfectly normal individuals. Everyone can observe a striking alteration of personality in others when they are exposed to varying conditions. A change from one environment to another is often enough to change the person into that other (mask) personality. Think about the *Lycopodium* child, that is a "house devil" (*speaks with an air of command, scolds much*) and "street angel" (*amativeness; child desires to be carried; feels frightened at everything, even ringing of a door bell*). Think about the *Silica* child, often rude and dictatorial at home, another "house devil" (*child becomes obstinate and when crossed has to restrain himself to keep from doing violence; very irritable, peevish mood*), but as soon as he sets foot in the world, he hides behind a family member (*yielding; faint-hearted; anxious mood; longing for his relations at home*).

—

So we can consider most people have "split" personalities, in other words, they easily dissociate into two main characters: the "social or professional character" and the "domestic" one. The social attitude (outward face) is governed by what is expected and dictated by society, as well as by the individual's motivations and ambitions (called "persona")[2]. The "domestic" character or inward face, on the other hand, is molded by emotional demands, which for a man are represented by the archaic soul image, the *anima*. This *anima* usually contains all those fallible human qualities his *persona* lacks. If the *persona* is intellectual (thinking function), the anima quite certainly will be sentimental (feeling function). Thus, many people have no "real" character; they are more a plaything of the circumstances, whereas the developed, balanced individual would respond with the same attitude and character no matter what the circumstances. This dissociation of character is even more visible in some professions. Consider the military person for instance. No matter what one's true individuality is and no matter what the military claims, it has little place for "individuals." One is expected to wear the accoutrements of a military professional. If someone behaves as an individual, it is rare for him to rise to high command; most will be dismissed as trouble makers, who will then blame the army for their failure in life. In reality, many of these people have continued down the unfortunate road they were forced to walk in their childhood when dominated by an authority figure. It is difficult for them to see that they have nourished and maintained their "chosen" life by joining a milieu that exactly reflects their sad childhood experience.

In striving to be more complete, we must continually pay attention to the symptoms arising from the unconscious contents and processes, in order to avoid a one-sided dominance of the consciousness. The most important function of the unconscious is trying to maintain homeostasis (a fine balance), but it certainly helps to keep this fine balance between consciousness and unconscious by a thorough and continued investigation of the unconscious in order to avoid getting stuck in blind alleys. It is this compensatory function that will allow the individual to avoid neuroses and psychotic breakdowns. We should avoid both repression and suppression and take advantage of the full investigation of both our worlds: the conscious and unconscious. We should keep in mind that the more civilized we are, the more we have a tendency to forget about the unconscious and the numerous undigested materials we have buried in it. Yet another

---

[2] *Persona*: A term introduced by Jung, referring to the masks worn by actors in the olden times. Persona involves not only the psychological qualities of a human being but also all forms of social behavior, habits of personal appearance (dress, hair style, etc.), facial expressions, manner of speaking, etc. It is part of the ego; the dominating function always rules the persona, while the inferior function has no part in it at all. For most people, though not for the true "individual," this persona is a mask. It serves to make an impression on others while concealing the true nature of the individual. Persona is like a geisha's make-up, hiding the true individual's features behind it.

reason to pay deliberate attention to that "invisible" other world, the unconscious, a world that can take on enormous proportions and overshadow our conscious if we neglect it.

Being more complete is taking that next step beyond becoming aware of the compensatory activity of the unconscious. At this point, we may feel fairly well adapted to the world in which we live, but we must feel compelled to go beyond the stage of adaptation or we will still remain a nameless face in the herds. The next step is becoming an individual, embarking on a spiritual journey, the process of individuation. Individuation is the psychological process that makes a human being an "individual", a unique unit or "whole man." Most of the great liberating deeds of the world's history originate from a leading personality like an *Aurum* or a *Sulphur*, and never from the masses. Becoming an individual is reaching for the gold in life; it is an act of high courage, a supreme realization, and the achievement of the greatest possible freedom that can be attained.

This also means paying a steep price, as isolation from the unconscious masses is inevitable. The battle to become an individual is therefore not such a popular undertaking, though people like *Aurum* and *Carcinosin* may have embarked on such a liberating path from childhood on. When in balance, they represent the seeds of the tree of humanity. Rather than following the beaten, easy path, they push forward into the narrow path leading to the unknown. Octavio Paz, who won the Nobel Prize in Literature in 1990, wonderfully expresses this idea:

> No one behind, no one ahead.
>
> The path the ancients cleared has closed.
>
> And the other path, everyone's path,
>
> Easy and wide, goes nowhere.
>
> I am alone and find my way.

What drives such people from a young age on? It is an inexplicable vocation, an irrational factor, almost a birth-right to be different from the masses. Such an individual is called by an inner voice and cannot resist that fate: it is a mandate he must obey. No doubt that *Aurum* involuntarily becomes a leader. In his assent to power, he will become a personality but can also succumb (the negative, syphilitic side) to the increasing load of responsibility, expressed by his numerous delusions (*lost affection of his friends*; *is unfit for this world*, etc.). But at least he has the opportunity to realize life's goal, becoming individualized. Most people fail in this mission but nature is merciful as it never puts the question, "Did you become an individual?" into people's mind. And so it goes: where no one asks, no one need tell.

The Danger of One Function Becoming Dominant

We cannot expect perfection, but too great a split in an individual between his thinking and feeling functions is dangerous. This, according to Jung, can already be called a slight neurosis, but it is not always to be viewed as negative! Every neurosis can be viewed as an attempt at self-cure, an attempt at compensation, and thus part of a self-regulating process; bringing out and further differentiating the inferior function can also be viewed as something positive. The secret is to pay attention to the process. This mechanism often achieves a better balance within the psyche. The neurosis is a warning and a call for help; as long as the ego is more or less intact, we can cure it through integrating conscious and unconscious contents, an interchange in which both sides must be put into shape to form a coherent Self, a psychological totality.

Of course, this integration of conscious and unconscious contents is a lifelong task, just as homeopathic treatment is a lifelong attempt to achieve or maintain homeostasis. This reflects the notion in homeopathy that every physical or emotional disease is an attempt by the body to cure itself: symptoms are the action of the patient's Vital Force (VF), which pushes signs to the exterior so we (patient and homeopath) can act on them! So, like physical diseases, neurosis with all its expressions is a friend rather than an enemy!

A neurosis can also develop if the naturally occurring dominant function is impeded (by circumstances, family, society, etc.), allowing the second or third function to take its place. At least there can never be a total atrophy of one of the functions; there is always a relative predominance of one type, never a "pure" type, just as there is no Yang without Yin and vice versa.

Some people think that this comfortable control by their main function protects them from any unfortunate psychological reaction, as though they could hide permanently in the safety of the dominant function. Mind you, this is what usually happens in this world! Such people forget the characteristic unreliability of the subordinate function (the shadow side) and the ease with which it can be influenced and escape from the dungeons. People often suffer from the delusion that mere suppression of the shadow side, the equivalent of cutting someone's head off to cure a headache, is adequate therapy. Depending on the situation, *Lycopodium's* normally superior thinking function can, for instance, be overwhelmed by his feelings, his "dark brother." And at that moment, *Lycopodium* could be classified as a feeling type. We are all familiar with the anticipation anxiety of *Lycopodium*, who, as a teacher, a lawyer, or a priest, is always well prepared (thinking function in superior position) but who can fall to pieces at the moment he has to deliver his message, overcome by anticipation anxiety and cowardice (the feeling function becoming the superior position). Characters like *Lycopodium* and *Silica* carry the greatest masks and hide behind their persona to survive, even thrive in their world. *Silica*, a "dominating" person in private, falls prey to his real Self and is overcome with timidity and bashfulness upon entering the world. Take, for example, a preacher: by day he is a powerful man, who through his thinking function mesmerizes the masses, yet at night, in his private life, this socially strong individual succumbs to his feelings, visiting sex workers and behaving like a child. Outwardly, this individual plays the role of a strong man; but at night he falls prey to his dark and untrained anima, since it is the anima that responds to the persona.

I had a friend who was psychologically injured by several poor relationships. He was predominantly in the introvert-thinking mode and could, to the despair of his new girlfriend, only express his feelings and vulnerability to his dog. "He kisses his dog all the time, while I have to ask for a kiss," she lamented. But when something trivial did not go his way (e.g., his girlfriend did not watch his whole tennis match), he would erupt in anger and spite: "I can never forgive you for not being there to support me during my match," he would exclaim.

It was obvious to me that when feeling became his dominant function, his reactions (to the amazement of his girlfriend) seemed grossly out of proportion. Of course, his underdeveloped function (feeling) is his shadow side and furiously tries to contain and guard his petty, antisocial, and frivolous qualities, but fails miserably when it is put to the test. This explained his moodiness and "childish" reactions in an otherwise seemingly well-controlled, guarded person. There was no acknowledgement on his part of this "foreign behavior," nor insight concerning it, to the despair of the feeling-type girlfriend. He acted later as though nothing had happened since he was now functioning again in his superior thinking function.

In this example, the overemphasized thinking function will set up compensation in the opposite (feeling) function, quite unexpectedly overwhelming the person with infantile reactions. In this example we can also clearly detect that most virile men have a feminine soul. Such an individual consciously denies his feminine traits and pushes them into his unconscious. This explains how my very virile friend could fall victim to his unconscious, feeling function (anima weakness).

I saw another extreme example of the thinking type with an almost non-existent feeling function on one of my travels. This person lived in another country separate from his wife and kids (made sense to him since his wife was making a lot of money), and, on the pretext of visiting his friend, my travel companion, he came to the city where we were staying. The real reason for his visit was to see his mistress in this city and my friend was just an excuse. When my unsuspecting friend found him in bed with the mistress (he was using our hotel room to "rest for a couple of hours"), he yelled at my friend to give him five minutes, whereupon he cold-bloodedly sent the lady friend away, as a used object, even though she had specifically interrupted a trip to another place to see him. He had no problems doing this (lack of feeling). He did not want to divorce his wife because that would cost him money, and although he was rather wealthy in his country, he would collect taxi fare receipts for 25 cents (thinking function) as a tax deduction!

He asked me whether there was something in homeopathy that could maintain his sexual drive forever. At the same time, he took a bossy and demeaning attitude towards the wait-staff in the restaurant (*dictatorial, speaking with a voice of command*). Any homeopath would love to give him *Lycopodium*! I foresee trouble in all his future relationships, even with his friends.

His wife was an intellectual, even more intelligent than he, so I foresee that the gap between them will only become wider. Jung explains that once that kind of man (a burnt-out *Lycopodium* in our homeopathic language) reaches a broken-down masculine lifestyle in his later life, he will then acquire some feminine or feeling characteristics (Campbell, 1976, p. 16). This is often accelerated by becoming ill and dependent on others (such as his wife). In the second half of her life, on the other hand, his thinking wife will develop more masculine tough-mindedness, further suppressing her inferior function of feeling. It is not hard to imagine that such a turn of events will lead to all sorts of problems in their marriage. As the husband discovers some feelings, and his wife increases her sharpness of mind the gap between them will increase. At the moment, neither has an inkling of such a transformation, and they are thus wholly unprepared to embark on the second half of their life's journey.

Compensation Between Extraversion and Introversion

Another reason for such tumultuous episodes is that there is always a compensatory relationship between extraversion and introversion. A *Sulphur* type may remain a successfully extraverted thinking type for a long time. Through the compensation process, such a consciously extraverted person has an introverted unconscious. I can remember how, right out of medical school, I was an extreme example of an extraverted thinking person, regarding psychology as a worthless sidebar of medicine. The lack of psychology instruction in our medical schools brainwashes countless physicians, making them believe that medicine is all science and no art. In critical moments, for instance, when a *Sulphur* loses the job where he thought he was irreplaceable, when his dominant function is muddled and loses control, the subjective elements in his unconscious will break loose and overwhelm his controlled behavior. Where before his dismissal, *Sulphur* was self-assured, optimistic, social, and generous, he now becomes censorious, avaricious, and egocentric. He feels misunderstood and withdraws like a hermit, transforming himself into a mal-adjusted introvert. A mal-adjusted *Sulphur* person, and other characters with delusions of grandeur (*Platina, Lycopodium, Lachesis, Veratrum album*), will also hide behind a frozen mask that obscures the deterioration of the individual. The rigid mask may be represented by identification with one's titles or office, as is often the case with politicians, professors, doctors, lawyers, etc. This might be an attractive mask, but behind it we would look in vain for substance. These are people who need to speak like a politician or a professor *all the time*: they don't differentiate when speaking to a child, their fiancée, or their business partner. They are not able to vary their persona as demanded by different situations; they have become one with their mask.

I had a patient who, when answering my question, "What brings you to me?" presented me with his curriculum vitae, which included all of his achievements. He had not come to apply for a job, but he had to reinforce his position with the importance alluded to in his papers: "I am a professor in such and such establishment," was the word. "Special" VIP treatment was therefore expected.

I remember, growing up in Belgium and practicing as a physician, how I was considered a rather "eccentric" and unusual individual since I did not conform to what was expected of me. Indeed, when I was dressed for tennis (on weekends, mind you) and appeared in a store, I could hear people whisper, "How can he be dressed like this, being a doctor!" If I was not imposing a persona on myself, the rest of Belgium was certainly trying hard to do so. This simply demonstrates that posing as someone (the mask!), doing what is expected by society according to one's professional status, is considered a virtue by most people. What such people don't realize, however, is that identification of their ego with the persona causes them to live a fallacy. Ask their wives, and you will get the real tale! The creation of such soulless individuals, according to the demands of society, appears to me to be self-sacrifice to an inferior public request. Blame my fondness for sports for my not playing the role assigned to me by public opinion! I wonder how this society would judge me now: I am a writer, teacher, physician, homeopath, acupuncturist, publisher, swimmer, tennis player, yoga adherent, and ballroom dancer. That surely makes me somewhat of a free thinker, an individual, which most often is either considered as upsetting the safety and "balance" of society where one is expected not to play more than one role, or being an eccentric whose views must somehow be considered unreliable: I could not possibly be all of these characters!

—

Chapter 11: The Eight Psychological Types

In Carl Jung's classification system, he defined eight psychological types: the introverted and the extraverted form of each type—thinking, feeling, sensation, and intuitive types. For instance, the extravert-thinking type (who has introverted feeling as his fourth and most primitive and undifferentiated side) rejects anything that depends on feeling and irrational phenomena, whereas the introvert-thinking type is less concerned with the facts but more with new views as he follows his own thinking inwards (introspection), ignoring criticism. Where the extravert-thinking type, with his bias toward the external world, is practical, the introvert-thinking type is impractical and has a disdain for publicity. Where extraverted-sensation types are guided by the object, introverted-sensation types are controlled by the subjective sensation the object causes.

Since introversion and extraversion are in and of themselves one-sided, the rule of compensation (at work also in dreams) requires, for a psychological balance, an unconscious counter-position. So an extraverted, intellectual person has an introverted feeling while an introverted-sensation type has an extraverted-intuitive side, and so on.

ATTITUDE & FUNCTION TYPES

Extravert Thinking

Introvert Sensation — Extravert Intuition

Introvert Feeling

We have already discussed the two attitude types in detail (Chap. 9). In this chapter we will take a closer look at the four function types with regard to their presence in homeopathy. Whether a function is differentiated or not is easily seen when people try to adapt themselves to different circumstances. If it is their strong point (well-differentiated) then this function is constant, stable, and something the person can put his trust in. Unfortunately, we usually have only one well-differentiated function, while the other three are often left in a

---

rather archaic mess. Let's have a closer look at the four functions and use this classification to understand and help our patient in his quest for self-realization.

The Thinking Type

Thinking Remedies in Homeopathy

Thinking is the function that seeks to understand the world and adjust to it by way of logical inferences: it entails the use of reason. The thinking type makes interpretative associations and gives more weight to thought when making important decisions. Whatever happens to them is subjected to consideration and reflection. People with a good mind (*Lachesis, Sulphur, Lycopodium, Aurum, China*, and *Sepia*) prefer to think, even *theorize*, about their situation. They can create theories for the sake of theories. The thinking type is very intellectual and dry and tries to force everything into a rationalistic system. He regulates his life according to straight lines and does not allow for anything related to feeling except perhaps the occasional concert (because it's appropriate for intellectuals to attend such functions). Thinking requires perception, reflection, and judgment and none of these characters have any deficit in that realm. **Sulphur**, the king of anti-psorics, will use his influential thought process in a passionate way: *he is greatly inclined to philosophical and religious reveries; very much excited and passionate; he racks his brains about metaphysical subtleties.* **China** (although an "artist" remedy) *has a desire for work, reading, writing, and reflecting; he has a general remarkable activity and industriousness. He has many ideas, and can build castles in the air. He makes many plans for the future and reflects upon their execution.* **Lachesis** *sits up late at night at mental work, with great activity and writes with the greatest vigor about everything he knows; new things constantly throng in his mind; increased power of originality in all mental work.* **Lycopodium** *has an excited, busy mood but changes from one subject to another, with difficulty of fixing the thought.* **Aurum**, *industrious and conscientious, is anxious to reflect deeply about this or that subject.* Note: Italic type denominates the language of Hering's materia medica, the source of the above text.

Feeling Function: Downfall of the Thinking Type

When thinking is superior and dominant, it goes without saying that the opposite function, *feeling*, will be in an inferior position. When you are intent on thinking clearly and with discernment, there is little room for feelings. One cannot possess two opposites in the same degree: this would go against the Law of Dissimilars (nothing can be more dissimilar than opposites). The stronger one suspends the weaker one (Aphorism 38). If it is to be real thinking, the person must scrupulously exclude feeling. In this case, the thinking person withdraws as much libido (psychic energy or force) as possible from the feeling process with the result that his feeling function becomes relatively unconscious and less exercised. The thinker is a highly conscious person, so firmly anchored in consciousness that nothing can pry him loose from it.

That does not mean that this type has no feelings. Au contraire! Eros or emotions for men are like rough diamonds that need to be polished. They are actually *afraid* of their emotions and often overcome by them. By all means, in all circumstances, they try to control their emotions through their intellect. A man usually counts it a virtue to repress his feelings, often considered to be a feminine weakness. What he does not know is that however hard he tries, he always will have the feminine (anima) in him, that soft emotional life. The anima also represents the serpent in paradise and is considered dangerous, magical, and taboo. If a high feeling-tone complex (in homeopathic language, a "Never Well Since" event linked to a very painful fixed emotion) is touched upon as by so little as a gesture or word, the high-strung thinking type can easily lose it.

In situations where the thinking type can only adapt through feeling, he will have to rely, to his despair, on his embryonic, archaic, and undeveloped inferior feeling function. This primitive feeling function gives rise to annoying outbursts and misunderstandings. The thinking type is forced to *accept* material from the inner world of the psyche, and once the inner adaptation is successfully achieved, a progression of the libido is again possible. This however takes *introspection*, which often is not possible. On Court TV, I saw a comment from a viewer regarding a murder case in which the perpetrator was a gifted academic. She formulated her remark: "For someone who is so academically gifted, he sure comes up short on common sense!" The preceding paragraphs provide the reader of this book with the explanation. In men, Eros, the function of love and relationships, is usually subservient to Logos, the "word or reason," while the reverse is often true for women. That's why men may have irrational moods and women irrational opinions.

Logic, reasoning, and objectivity are characteristics that usually belong to the ideal male's outward attitude or persona (especially in the thinking function), characteristics in which he finds support at all times. Such a man easily falls prey to melancholia, to despair, and even to suicide. With women we have the opposite. Their outward attitude is ideally that of feeling, so they always find comfort and hope as they can recall their inner voice, their reasoning when necessary.

Take for example someone who has been dominated from childhood to adulthood. He finally decides to stand up for himself (*Carcinosin* state) and not betray his true self anymore. He is pleased that he feels in control now, especially after reading many self-help books, perhaps even more advanced books like Jung's. But when his wife inadvertently, through an innocent gesture or phrase, touches upon his very sensitive feeling complex (ailments from domination), he bursts out in an avalanche of furious anger. The thinking function now plays second fiddle to the feeling function. To an outsider, not knowing the whole story, this reaction seems to be blown out of all proportion. After the storm is over, the thinking type resumes his previous position and is disappointed and perplexed at how he, an "intelligent" being who takes pride in his stiff upper lip could stumble so quickly and unexpected. He thought he was full of feeling but in reality it is just sentimentality; he has no feeling because he is all mind. Sentimentality, in this case, is a weakness, and always a sign of inferior feeling. It never fails that *Sulphur* patients tell me how much they are in touch with their feelings: "Dr Luc," they say, "I cry at the movies! I must be full of feelings because my tears flow easily." As the person gets older, this sentimentality manifests itself ever more easily.

The difference between a feeling and thinking type is most patent when, for example, a person of one kind is the partner (business or marriage) of a person of the other type. I once treated a retired attorney who took up tap dancing with some of his buddies, after having lived in a world of constant "power-thinking." At first this interest in dancing made it appear that he was exploring his "feeling attitude," something he had neglected till then. Much effort was put into his tap dancing performance—costumes, regular rehearsals, etc. At their first performance in a bistro, not many people paid attention, and he was quite annoyed. Although he thought he had tapped into his "feeling function," his dominant function remained "thinking" (which could easily be seen in the hard work he put into the preparation of his performance). He wanted to garner praise for this performance as he had as a lawyer. Speaking of delusions of grandeur: he even had thoughts of "touring the US"! He was driving his wife crazy, infringing on her terrain—her home life, since he wanted to micro-manage everything with his superior thinking. His wife could hardly stand it and probably would have liked to see him go on tour!

Real marital problems begin for such people when a misunderstanding arises. They put all the blame on their spouse because he possesses qualities that, in him, are in a very undifferentiated and inferior form. This can happen in any sort of relationship: between friends, parents and children, boss and subordinates, and yes, between the homeopath and his patient! Here again, the concerned party (homeopath included) needs to explore and develop his opposite, inferior function type (feeling in this case), which would go a long way toward helping him become more balanced and also more understanding of the other person.

—

Most of the above-mentioned "thinking" remedies struggle with that dual aspect (thinking-feeling). The dominant intellectual side can be overcome in some circumstances by feelings that are archaic, primitive, and undeveloped: it surprises most everyone how very intellectual people can act as complete fools when it comes to love affairs and women. The inferior feeling side of the thinking type is also no match for the individual with a high feeling tone; just look around and you see many *Sulphur* types (the thinking type) married to *Phosphorus* people (the feeling type; see further). The undoing of the thinking type, his Achilles tendon, is his feelings. No wonder so many of these *Sulphur* types and others regard feelings as dangerous and frivolous, to be avoided at all cost. In my practice, I often heard the feeling type, *Phosphorus* wife, complain about the insensitivity of her *Sulphur* husband. She does not know that this conduct is a must for the *Sulphur* in order to stay "at the top of his game" with his goal clearly in mind: becoming famous! For that, he needs to be in control of his life. So here is a piece of advice for the *Phosphorus* woman: never force the intellectual *Sulphur* into his feelings! He knows he cannot be attacked in his intellect, and he does not want his weak flank (his feelings) exposed. He will rule his feelings with an iron fist, lest they make him lose control!

Thinking and Feeling: Always Different in Intensity

Here we have yet another confirmation that thinking and feeling cannot exist at the same time in the same intensity, even though we may strive for that end. The content of this feeling-tone complex (an unresolved emotion to which the person is now addicted) most often disappears from the conscious mind and is deposited in the unconscious or shadow side, from where it can come back to haunt the person. Don't forget that this emotion can be transferred intrauterine, "infecting" the unborn fetus with his mother's core delusion (CD). The child will show all kinds of behavior, reminiscent of the mother's feelings, as the unborn fetus was susceptible to the mother's emotions. In this shadow world, the ego is somewhat dark, and we can always discover something new about ourselves. But just like delusions, this feeling-toned memory complex (our homeopathic NWS), hidden from view in the unconscious, can still lead to certain actions as if it were present in the conscious mind, when called up through minor gestures or words. We have to remember that the greater part of all our psychic elements (the "real" us versus the mask) resides in the unconscious, cast out of our conscious as not to disturb some of our delusional thoughts, or more simply not to ruffle our illusionary life, in which we desire to be someone other than the person we *are*.

In the case of children, and even of adults who remain stuck, the unconscious part of the psyche offers a degree of safety. In order to be functional in life, more or less rational, the unconscious must harbor untold psychological complexes; in other words, it is the dumping ground of anything that we don't like or fear.

When the control of the conscious mind is lifted, the voice of the unconscious, dreams, can tell us the craziest stories. "I dreamed of you with another woman," the exasperated wife might say. "What does it mean," she asks? If anything, it refers to those insecure thoughts she suffered when she herself cheated on her fiancée. It has nothing to do at all with her present husband, but only reflects her own "devious" animus. Most of us, even saints, would not want to divulge those horrifying sexual exploits we commit in dreams. Even St. Augustine asked God to forgive him for his dreams. The unconscious remains the "master," (the "real" us) which, especially when there is an *"abaissement du niveau mental"* (a lowering of the mental level as seen in neuroses, delusions, and psychosis), can inundate and confuse its "slave," the conscious mind, resulting in numerous delusions, that may begin to dictate actions and thoughts.

As we saw in the previous example, the brain never seems to forget the slightest impression, which often leaves more than a trace in the memory. If that same impression is repeated over time, it can create fearful fixed ideas, as the impressions occupy more and more space in our memory bank.

I read in some advisory column an example of the thinking type. It was "an ultra responsible young man", who graduated from college with honors, landed a lucrative job with a stable company, and had a lot of friends and a girlfriend.

"His present 'problem' is that he takes life too seriously. He says he is the cerebral type. He analyzes, intellectualizes, and evaluates almost everything he does. He does not laugh a lot and can't seem to have fun. These shortcomings in his character, he says further, have caused problems in his relationships."

It is obvious that this young man has never explored his primitive side as he probably, at the age of 22, has just firmly established his thinking function, and it is the tool he feels comfortable with in his approach to the world. Of course, the feeling types of his age (the ladies) will be turned off by this "boorish intellectual" behavior. For entirely different reasons, *Arsenicum, Aurum,* and *Natrum sulphuricum* (remedies that might be helpful in the above case) score high for the rubrics: *seriousness; responsible and early responsibility;* and *industriousness.*

Feeling Equals Thinking

The only instance where feeling and thinking are equal in intensity is in primitive people and young children, where consciousness and unconsciousness are uniform. What a primitive man experiences in a dream is just as real to him as what he sees when he is awake. Both thinking and feeling occur to a relatively undeveloped degree. Just like in the first developmental stage of the child (in general the first two years), the consciousness of the primitive man is still uncertain, still in a state of unsteady gait and vertigo, so to speak. In very young children and primitive people, the four functions remain undifferentiated. Where normally the differentiation should be finished by the end of adolescence, some people never achieve enough differentiation to wrest themselves away from childhood. I refer to the elements of the Periodic Table, which I have called the "dependent" remedies in the second group from Level II to Level VI (*Magnesium, Calcarea, Strontium, Baryta*). A perfect example is *Baryta carbonica*, who has the CD, *his legs are cut off and he walks on his knees*. This delusion expresses a lack of confidence and the high need for support, especially from family or close friends. *Baryta carbonica* is *even* listed in the rubric: *childish behavior in old age*. A *Baryta carbonica* person is certainly the one where differentiation of the four types has been at a minimum, leaving him an insecure and vulnerable person for most of his life. Children initially need to discover their dominant function and attitude type before they can explore the opposite ones later in life. One-sidedness not only threatens to create neuroses or even psychosis, it also hinders a person's individuation process and also any relationship he will have with others.

In primitive people, as well as children, the contents of the individual psyche are not yet differentiated from those of the collective psyche. Therefore, just like young children, it is very easy for primitive people to be invaded by the unconscious in the form of archetypal dreams. Jung had examples in his practice where a young child could not liberate herself from her archetypal dream and died a year later. In his words, this reflected that "she was never born." This shows the danger of the powerful, often fearsome archetypal image for which primitive people have the greatest respect, fearing they might become possessed by it. This uncontrolled emotion washes over the primitive person (or child) like a big wave, making him do things that are strange to him. These archetypal images constitute their "big" dreams. As a defense mechanism, from ancient times, people have invented all kinds of purification rites to save the soul. These are still the basis of much of what religion stands for.

Equally dangerous, I think, is trying to integrate unconscious contents into consciousness in young children who have buried unpleasant events in their unconscious. I was confronted with this possibility on my trip with Homeopaths Without Borders, as we offered homeopathic help to tsunami victims. I read about the foreign psychotherapists in Sri Lanka, trying, after one month of counseling, to get children to recount their memories through drawings and discussions. They tried to force subconscious contents to become one with the conscious. While this goal is laudable and necessary, since suppression of the unconscious contents can only lead to neurosis, even psychosis. So the speed at which this process should be done must be customized to the individual. We must take into account the temperament, constitution, and active miasm, and yes, the collective unconscious of the Sri Lankan people, their customs, and habits.

Therefore, looking at the sum of the conscious and unconscious (the source of dreams and the CD) serves as the basis for selecting a homeopathic remedy that can make the healing process faster, more gentle, and permanent, as promised in Aphorism 2 of the *Organon*.

Forcing the child to recollect the horrors of the tsunami when she is not ready, not strong enough to face the horror again (and this because the therapist is driven by time constraints), is a threatening event for the child and exposes her to a dark force that can be quite overwhelming. When you are not ready for freedom, it feels just like prison.

The children in the Sri Lankan experiment did not have the patience to sit still and draw pictures expressing their tsunami experience. I wonder if these children were unconsciously resisting the forced attempt at integrating these unconscious contents with the conscious, if they did not instinctively sense the danger of such procedure. I know that this process of drawing is similar to what Jung did with his patients, getting them to paint their feelings and emotions. But these young children have no dominant function as yet so this integrating process, if not exercised *individually* (each at their own speed), could overwhelm the conscious, causing delusions, neuroses, and, yes, even psychotic breaks. Hence, the prime importance and necessity of homeopathic treatment of such young tsunami victims, which must, in and of itself, be individualized.

The Negative Side of the Homeopathic Thinking Type

The previously mentioned characters (*Sulphur, Lachesis, Aurum, Lycopodium,* and *China*) will use their thoughts and intellect to dull their CD by planning, researching, reading avidly, discussing, attending support groups, studying, reflecting, debating, theorizing, etc. These tactics help them stay on the pathway of positive compensation. Inevitably, in so doing, they will suspend their feeling values because this is the only way they can think in a firm, dispassionate way. They equate feelings and sensitivity to being irrational, thus a hindrance to logical scientific and philosophical thought. As a result, they can often be capricious, irritable, censorious, patronizing, domineering socially, overbearing know-it-alls, seemingly in control of their feelings like the good old English chap, but in reality, terribly bothered by their feelings. Sooner or later they will have to face the music and listen to their feelings. Often this will bring them to the negative, destructive path with the formation of secondary delusions. Let's see what this means for some of the thinking types.

For **Sulphur**, a time always comes, especially upon retirement, when the audience for his philosophical ranting is missing: as a result he suffers from *melancholic moods, dwells on religious and philosophical speculations with anxiety about his soul's salvation* and he shows *indifference about the lot of others*. Aurum's intellectual efforts and industriousness at some point become vain and fail to be appreciated; turning him into an individual *who imagines that he is unfit for this world, and longs for death with internal delight, since he lost the affection of his friends.* Lycopodium suffers *vexation* and *cannot endure the slightest contradiction or opposition and becomes overpowered by many unpleasant recollections.* He has *dreams of his boat foundering* and *fears that he cannot reach his destination.* In other words, his CD, *he has done wrong and everything will vanish*, comes true. **Lachesis** ultimately *becomes easily peevish and mistrustful and believes himself intentionally injured by his environment* (his CD), *attaching the most hateful significance to the most innocent occurrences.* **China** feels that everyone is out to obstruct his ambitions and plans (*thinks he is hindered and tormented by everyone*) and *now seeks every opportunity for being angry.* As we can see, the thinkers appear to be "unfeeling," but in reality they are protective of their feelings and accomplish this by suppressing their feelings. Eventually this will lead to an array of negative emotions, destructive in nature, when feelings are unleashed from the unconscious into the conscious.

The Feeling Type

Defining Feeling

Feeling and sensation are often confused in English but are more clearly differentiated in the French language with the words, "sentiment" and "sensation." Feeling (sentiment) regulates thinking: the laws of logic, reflection, and judgment are suspended in favor of the aims of feeling. The feeling person understands the world by evaluating her feelings: "pleasant or unpleasant, acceptable or unacceptable, beautiful, ugly, happy, sad, etc." "My feeling about this is such and such," she says. But "feeling" is still considered a rational function as it still uses judgment and evaluation. Feeling people neglect thinking in favor of emotional factors: they follow a policy dictated by feeling, and it takes an extraordinary situation for them to reflect before acting.

The **extravert**-feeling type is found mainly in women whose feelings are based on external things. For them, a suitable husband is one who earns enough money to give them a luxurious lifestyle and satisfy their compulsive pleasure-seeking behavior (*Phosphorus*) or desire for status (*Platina*). The **introvert**-feeling type shows interest in the subject (the Self) and tends to look for ways to explore it: yoga, meditation, psychological studies, etc. Jung includes moral feeling as well as other kinds of sentiment such as love, compassion, empathy, and tenderness in the feeling type.

When feeling is the dominant function, thinking is necessarily in an inferior position. Musicians, painters, artists of all kinds often can't think at all, because they never intentionally use their brains. When such a person wants to feel (deeply and purely), "thinking" must be downplayed as much as possible. It is obvious that we cannot possess two opposite states in the same degree of perfection, although some people claim they have perfected both to the same degree. This is analogous to what we see in homeopathic constitutions: one can see, for example, that someone is mainly *Sulphur* (superior or dominant) with a small part of *Phosphorus* (inferior condition). A person cannot be a 100 percent *Sulphur* and a 100 percent *Phosphorus*! That is not to say that the feeling type cannot think! But he will approach Logos from the point of Eros, formulating it as, "I cannot express things that I don't feel!" Of course life is full of ever-changing feeling situations, changeable moods like those we see in *Phosphorus* and *Pulsatilla*, two feeling types.

If the feeling type allows himself to be disturbed by thoughts, he easily falls under their spell, and they become delusions: he is imprisoned by these thoughts. Delusional thoughts become immovable (delusions **are** fixed ideas) in which the feeling type gets caught up. A perfect example are the many delusions of the deeply empathetic and oversensitive *Phosphorus*: he sees all kinds of ghosts, animals, spirits, faces, devils, shadows, and is easily overwhelmed by them. Because of their vivid imagination, thinking can be dangerous for the feeling type.

These are equally intelligent people who simply find their way by feeling, not thinking. Feeling is an entirely subjective process. It can be a kind of judging but it does not establish an intellectual connection between the ego and a given content. The only aim is to award a value, to accept or reject it. Feeling types are considered good social mixers, artists, and creative people. They are empathetic and live and die by their feelings. They seem to possess a more natural relationship with the unconscious. That does not mean that every artist will derive benefit from producing an eye-catching work, fished from his or her unconscious. She must not only explore such images, but also understand the symbolic language this work represents. I knew a great artist who tapped into her unconscious to produce the most amazing but dark paintings. She operated best under the influence of alcohol and at night, which made it easier to connect to her unconscious. Alas! Her conscious life was such a wreck, with alcoholism ruling her life, that her fogged brain could not integrate the messages released from the unconscious with the conscious. Her paintings had artistic value, but her work was an incomplete psychological event, and she was unable to further her individuation process by painting such "dark" pieces.

It is easy to confuse emotion with feeling. Jung calls emotion an affect, triggered by an active, often painful complex. This affect has a tendency to distort each of the four existing functions and here we find the confusion. Indeed, when we are mad or sad, we can't think logically. When we are overly happy, we judge people incorrectly, and when we are depressed, we can't tap into our intuition.

Feeling Types in Homeopathy

I deviate here from what Jung termed "feeling" in his extravert and introvert types. Jung's understanding of feeling was more a value judgment, "Does this feel agreeable, good, bad, etc.?" Or he refers to the French word, "sentiment," which can be an attitude but can also be translated in the sense of, "It is the feeling (sentiment) of this group that we will support that candidate," referring to an **opinion**.

For us homeopaths, in order to know **who** these people are, we look at rubrics reflecting "sensitivity." One place to find the analogy with feeling in homeopathy is in the rubric: *sensitive, oversensitive*. This can be linked to sensitive when hearing of cruelty (*Calcarea carbonica, Phosphorus, Carcinosin*); sensitive children (mainly *Carcinosin, Pulsatilla, Phosphorus, Ignatia,* and *Staphysagria*); sensitive to the arts (*Carcinosin*); sensitive to criticism (**Carcinosin**, *Staphysagria*); sensitive to all external impressions (**Phosphorus**, *Staphysagria, Carcinosin*); sensitive to being laughed at (*Calcarea carbonica*); sensitive to moral impressions (*Staphysagria, Ignatia*); sensitive to reprimands (*Ignatia, Calcarea carbonica*); and sensitive to rudeness (**Staphysagria**, *Calcarea carbonica, Carcinosin*). Of course, we have many more remedies (*Medorrhinum,* the *Natrums,* etc.) but *Carcinosin, Phosphorus, Calcarea carbonica, Ignatia,* and *Staphysagria* seem to be outstanding remedies, which could be classified under Jung's feeling types. We could also refer to "hysterical" behavior as subgroup of the feeling type: for example, *Ignatia* and its chronic complement, *Natrum muriaticum.* We see clearly that when the patient is in a full-blown state of grief related to *Natrum muriaticum,* she easily loses control as the thinking function (and judgment) undergoes an "*abaissement,*" a lowering or decreasing. Now we understand why *Natrum muriaticum* can be overcome with hatred and vindictiveness, as seen in the provings, *although evidently a well-educated and intelligent woman, her mind seemed hopeless and confused.* In cases of grief, the bigger picture of *Natrum muriaticum,* which is *Sepia,* with a clear thinking-function (to the point of exhaustion and ailments from mental overwork), is pushed into a latent state and plays second

—

fiddle to *Natrum muriaticum*. The practical, business-like achiever, *Sepia*, loses the battle when the patient slips into a *Natrum muriaticum* state after a betrayal or a deception.

Compensations Used by the Feeling Type

How does the feeling type fare on the pathways of compensation and destruction? Depending on the remedy picture, the feeling type will use social strengths, sympathy, caring, an overly active sense of responsibility, and love for humankind and especially animals, to stay on the positive pathway. How long he can hold out all depends on his tenacity, stubbornness, and unfortunately, the betrayal of his own soul. Eventually, because of exhaustion on all planes (*Phosphorus*), because of constant suppression by others (*Staphysagria*), because of self-imposed high expectations (*Carcinosin*), or because of an under-developed ego (*Calcarea carbonica*), the "stress" they experience will bring them towards a negative and destructive pathway. Let's take a closer look at some of these personalities and see if we can find the dominance of feeling over thinking in the provings for the outspoken feeling remedies—*Phosphorus, Calcarea carbonica, Staphysagria,* and *Carcinosin*.

Phosphorus—The Vata Type in Ayurvedic Medicine

Certainly *Phosphorus* with *an excited imagination has an overactive mind*, but because of the dominant feeling-tone, *has difficulties arranging this great flow of thoughts*. The dominant feeling value easily can be found in the many delirium expressions of *Phosphorus*, not surprisingly also found in the sexual sphere: *this delirium was erotic, with great indications of the sexual system; delirium with fear of death; delirium with constant attempts to escape; delirium with fearful cries, striking, and biting*, etc. The other side of the coin, the thinking value, is, as expected, primitive: *great indisposition to mental or physical exertion; disinclination to study; inability to think; could not study nor keep his mind on any particular subject long at a time*. These symptoms are all graded in the highest degree. Not surprisingly, in Hering's provings of *Phosphorus* he discusses ailments from disappointed love, and describes the symptom: a *crazy delirium in a young woman who was strictly moral and unhappy in her love; she accused herself of the most obscene actions, of which she never was guilty.*

Carcinosin

We have here a very fragile person who undermines his own confidence by pleasing others while suppressing his own wishes. It is their desire for harmony in family and the world with an acutely felt connection to suffering that will eventually be their downfall. The rigidity and high expectations in the upbringing of *Carcinosin* leave him with a heavy legacy. Every choice in life, every task or performance, carries with it a life or death sentence. His over-developed sense of duty and commitment creates an overburdened seriousness that leads him to worry about every decision that he makes. This will lead to consulting the homeopath and psychotherapist when he has lost the ability to continue to make decisions: his feeling function is so strong that thinking, which is necessary to make meaningful decisions, is reduced to a minimal state. The attempt to maintain order and definition in his life overwhelms him to the point that he can no longer move forward! Even when coming into adulthood, he sets himself up for situations that demand incredibly high standards.

The *Carcinosin* child is often created as a result of being given early responsibility. If you **expect** a child to grow up very quickly, then the opposite often happens to the child's feeling about himself. It is very likely that the child will be able to take responsibility for the household, but he will not have been given the time and freedom to explore himself through the normal process of growing up and experiencing childhood and adolescence. Children and teenagers form their sense of who they are through reacting to authority and to the constraints of society. In the expanse of their personality they find their ego. They may be forced into this situation because one of the parents has died, for instance, the mother in which case the oldest daughter takes on her role, or the parent is unable to parent effectively because of illness or drug addiction. It can be as benign as the parents demanding that the oldest child be a perfect example for the younger ones to follow. Any of these situations may force the child to grow up quickly, perhaps even taking responsibility for running the household.

Obviously, great expectations are put on the *Carcinosin* individual, not only by others but also by himself. Failure in any task is just not acceptable and is tantamount to not receiving love and validation from others and the self. This pressure undermines his self-confidence and leads to irresolution as he is overburdened by high expectations. No wonder that anticipation anxiety is a fixed trait of *Carcinosin*. To avoid quarrels and criticism, he does not put up boundaries and gives in to everything, neglecting his own desires and wishes. In a sense, he betrays himself, making statements like, "I can't say no; I hate confrontations; I feel guilty when I take time off; I am not allowed to fail." This also leads to a great deal of suppressed anger, which eventually leads to physical illness. In his more lucid moments, he will say, "The greatest injustice is that I am never accepted the way I am." Keep in mind that *Carcinosin, Causticum,* and *Staphysagria* are intimately connected to each other.

Calcarea carbonica—The Kapha Type in Ayurvedic Medicine

Calcarea carbonicum's sensitive feeling tone strikes a different chord from that of *Phosphorus* and *Carcinosin*. The feeling function is in a superior position only because the *Carbon* person remains stuck in his individuation process. While *Carcinosin* and *Phosphorus* are "black-type" remedies under the rubric—*sympathetic*—*Calcarea carbonica* is only graded a 1! Their sympathy does not carry further than their own family (*affections from egotism*), which leads to a sensitivity that is linked to any threat to their personal safety (home, immediate family, and health). It is indeed revealing that *Calcarea carbonica's* sensitivity is best expressed in the rubric, *sensitive to hearing bad news and sad stories.* Her vivid imagination easily conceives of dangers: *mind full of concern about imaginary things that might happen to her; she thinks and talks of nothing but murder, fire, rats, etc.; fears that something sad and terrible will happen to her. Frightened, apprehensive mood, as if some misfortune were about to happen to him, or someone else, which he could in no way overcome.* No wonder, *she desires to go home, look for company,* and has a *great desire to be mesmerized.* Her sensitivity is also linked to the way people view her and talk to her: *easily offended; takes everything amiss; weeps when admonished.* Weeping comes easily, another hallmark of her sensitive character: *weeping about trifles, with a sensitive, irritable mood. Despondent and melancholic, in the highest degree, with a kind of anguish.* We can see that the thinking function is in an inferior position by studying the proving symptoms: *thinking is difficult; intellect dull; unable to progress in her studies; mind is confused, so that what is read or heard is not understood or comprehended; appears to be lapsing into complete imbecility; the slight effort of talking gave him sensation as if the brain would be paralyzed, mostly in the occiput.* We can see how easily confused this individual becomes: anything slightly demanding brings her into a panic. She is convinced that *she will lose her reason,* or that *people will observe her confusion of mind.* Obviously, fears, anxieties, and worries about very personal matters are often the cause of their sensitive reactions: *fright followed by trembling motions of upper and lower limbs in repeated paroxysms.*

Staphysagria

The central idea of *Staphysagria* is *suppression of the emotions and pent-up wrath or anger.* Like so many of us, *Staphysagria* is the victim of her expectations and desires, especially those revolving around relationships. Belonging to Jung's "sensitive type," the sentimental *Staphysagria* has an outspoken naiveté when it comes to relationships. She thinks everyone is like her but she receives a rude awakening when reality sets in. Rather than openly expressing her anger as does *Nux vomica* or *Sulphur, Staphysagria* will resort to resignation and submissiveness.

Because her indignation finds no natural outlet, she swallows her wrath. She is too dignified to fight (delusions: *of humility of others while she is great; suffering from pride, envy or chagrin*). *Staphysagria* becomes ill from the conflicts around her (*great indignation about things done by others or by himself; grieves about consequences*). So *Staphysagria's* sensitivity revolves around the most innocent impressions. More than anyone else she suffers from rudeness, vexation, and reserved displeasure (*very sensitive to the least impression; least word that seems wrong hurts her very much*). Unkind words or actions from her husband and children easily hurt her feelings: *every word vexes her; she cries even if one only speaks to her.* *Staphysagria* is so sensitive that when she has to control herself, she goes to pieces and trembles from head to foot, loses her voice, loses her ability to work, cannot sleep—all followed by a headache. *She grieved over her condition and wept: nothing in the world pleased her.* Although we are talking about pent-up anger, often *Staphysagria* expresses *partial* anger: *very peevish; he wishes to throw from him everything which he takes in his hand.*

The thinking sensation becomes inferior (*inability to think; has no desire to think, he is mentally exhausted*) as this person becomes numb and paralyzed: vanishing of thoughts when interrupted in conversation (also *Thuja*)—*on attempting to grasp an idea, it vanishes; thoughts disappear whenever he attempts to think or speaks of any subject;* and *if anyone interrupts him or changes to another subject, he, for the moment, forgets, or cannot at all collect his thoughts. He is indisposed to serious work: a few minutes after reading anything, he forgets everything; he is scarcely able to recall it after a long reflection; want of memory with heavy weight between the eyes.*

The Intuitive Type

Defining Intuition

Intuition comes from the Latin, *intueri*: to look into or upon. This psychological function transfers perceptions in an **unconscious** way, which excludes the cooperation of sensation. We say that intuitive people have a sixth sense for hidden possibilities. Unconscious perception of the possibilities inherent in a situation, unduly influenced by existing reality, defines the intuitive type. Intuition is a kind of perception that cannot be traced directly to conscious sensory experience. It is instinctive understanding where pure intellect cannot understand: its irrational nature does not easily allow rational judgment and investigation. The intuitive type "knows" things without the need for reasoning. Intuition is similar to *instinct*, the inborn manner of acting: the homeopath perceives many things in his patient that he could never obtain through a purely intellectual approach. "I feel intuitively that this mission is going to be a success." It is an unconscious "inner perception." Intuitive processes are spontaneous, dynamic and bewilderingly devious. There is no use in rationalizing and intellectualizing this activity.

The primary function of intuition is to transmit images and conditions which could not be gained by the other functions or only by very roundabout ways, since the other functions—thinking, feeling, and sensation—are more or less suppressed. Sensation, in the opposite position, is naturally most affected as it disturbs the naïve, instinctive, and unbiased awareness of the intuition. The intuitive person possesses sensations, but they do not guide him. In this function, conclusions are not drawn from content; conclusions are drawn in a seemingly irrational way because the intuitive person doesn't seem to be able to explain how he came to those conclusions. Intuition is the instrument which, in the presence of a hopelessly blocked situation, works automatically towards a solution that no other function could discover.

Yet persons with superior intuition have a great degree of conviction concerning their intuitive cognition, unless thinking is their secondary function, which can impose a need for an explanation. Like any irrational type, the intuitive states striking judgments and coldhearted criticisms (*censorious, intolerance*), which may have the stamp of naiveté, but, at times, can be inconsiderate, crude, and outrageous (*rudeness, fanaticism, impatience*).

Who Is This Person?

The **extravert**-intuitive type is your typical tubercular person: he feels a great need for change because of lingering dissatisfaction; stable conditions suffocate him. This is the typical enthusiastic beginner, but bad finisher, as a newer and "more exciting" prospect has showed up before he gets to the end of a project. "What happened to your dream of becoming a real estate broker?" "Oh, that was two months ago," the intuitive-extravert answers after some thought. That was an "old" project! Now she is totally absorbed by this new opportunity, and the rest of her life has conveniently vanished! Even their moods change from one moment to another: just yesterday, that boyfriend was her soul mate, today he is her suffocating nightmare! In this type, thinking or feeling, are subordinate functions and carry almost no weight in the decision-making process. The intuitive type lacks the ability to make thoughtful judgments.

Intuition rules and no thinking or feeling can lead her away from this new relationship or enterprise: "My intuition tells me, he's the right guy!" Or, "It's the right opportunity to make money!" Past failures don't count, as the intuitive powers squash any reasonable approach with brutal force. These are the women who exploit social situations: making the right social connections, marrying the guy with money or political influence and power. These are the women who, because their husbands support them financially, have the *delusion of doing business*.

The extravert-intuitive male will look for professions in fields where his intuition can guide him: politics, exploration, and the stock market are attractive to this type. Often, when they have more altruistic goals in mind, they may become a very positive factor economically and socially. Their unbridled enthusiasm, even short-lived, might be enough to ignite the flame of a great enterprise. As long as there are others, more of the thinking or even sensation type, to continue the brilliant inspirational moments of the intuitive, all is not lost. I was, for example, the benefactor of the great intuitive powers of my wife, Yolanda, when she chose my secretary among 20 candidates. I have never had a better one!

Since the intuitive type can't stay put, others often profit from her open, willing, and enthusiastic nature. Because she lacks stamina, she eventually burns out after everyone has taken advantage of her. Staying put is just not in her character! Since thinking and feeling are often archaic and infantile in this person, the intuitive may project intense phobias (the archaic feeling) such as we find in *Phosphorus*.

Of course, the feeling and thinking types can have intuition as a supporting function and vice versa. So we see prophetic dreams in *Sulphur* and *Aconite* and mesmerizing qualities in *Lachesis, Silica, Calcarea carbonica*, and *Phosphorus*.

The **introvert**-intuitive type is the grotesque and whimsical artist, the mystic, the visionary, or the misunderstood genius, which can be *China* or the burnt-out *Sulphur*.

According to Jung, fastidious types prefer intuition. In homeopathy, these would include: *Arsenicum, Nux vomica*, and the *Kali* remedies, the most outspoken being *Kali arsenicum*.

In order to find the homeopathic remedies related to intuition, I looked at the following rubrics found mostly in the *Mind* section (characteristics expressed by Jung):

CHARACTERISTICS OF THE INTUITIVE

- Censorious
- Clairvoyant
- Dictatorial, talking with air of command
- Fanatic
- Impatient
- Impulsive
- Indifferent, does not complain
- Intolerant
- Intuitive
- Irrational
- Prophetic dreams
- Rudeness
- Sensitive

—

The leading remedies in these rubrics (taken in order of importance according to the function in the Radar software program, "Sum of symptoms and degrees"):

1. *Sulphur* 24

2. *Nux vomica* 23

3. *Phosphorus* 21

4. *Lycopodium* 20

5. *Aconite* 19

6. *Lachesis* 19

7. *Arsenicum* 17

Among all the above remedies, we see clearly that the thinking types (*Sulphur, Lycopodium, Nux vomica, Lachesis*) use intuition as a secondary function. Only three feeling types, *Phosphorus, Aconite* (the restless, frightened individual), and *Arsenicum* (the nervous race horse), score high in the intuitive function. *Phosphorus*, when in a feeling-intuitive state, has no boundaries, there are no closed doors and no inhibitions, and she can sense and experience everything without the function of sensation—*as if in a dream.*

The Sensation Type

Defining Sensation

This *irrational,* perceptive function is like intuition. Sensation tells us that something *is,* but it does not tell us *what* it is. Sensation perceives things as they are. Sensation operates with perceptions that are not evaluated or interpreted; therefore the sensation function is irrational. Thinking will tell us what an object is. If you are the sensation type, then your favored way of relating to reality is via physical sensation. Sensation not only concerns outer stimuli but also inner ones, as we can perceive sensations related to diseased organs. Sensation is not the same as feeling; the former is a *sensory perception*, where the latter is a *judgment.*

Take the example of watching a sunset: it is not only the image of the sun setting, but also the perception of multiple colors and forms that often evokes feelings of peacefulness, romanticism, or being at one with the earth. The **sensation** type will note each detail of this lovely scene: the colors of the sky and the sun, cloud formations, birds, airplanes, people in the distance, etc. The **intuitive** type, on the other hand, will pay very little attention to detail but will be overwhelmed by the general atmosphere of beauty and serenity. *Abstract* sensation, on the other hand, focuses on only one aspect of this natural phenomenon: on the radiating, intensely bright orange color, for instance. No other aspect is part of the content of our consciousness, and we remain entirely detached from all the other aspects mentioned before. This abstract sensation seems to be best suited to the artist.

Sensation is the most prominent function in children and primitive people as they explore their surrounding world mainly through their senses. The **sensation** type is the fact-minded person, for whom judgment, feeling, and intuition take on a secondary importance. The sensation type hears the words sounding in his ears, he sees the things before his eyes, and he notices the things he touches or tastes. Many intelligent people live as though they had never learned to use their sense organs. In the sensation type, sensation definitely dominates the thinking and feeling functions, but not necessarily intuition. **Intuition is an unconscious perception while sensation is a conscious perception.** Normal sensations are proportionate to the intensity of the physical stimulus. An exaggerated, abnormally strong sensation occurs when the dominant function sensation blends with a still undifferentiated other function (thinking, feeling, sexual) as we can see in the **carbon level** of the Periodic Table.

The **extravert**-sensation type is the typical *Carbon* pleasure-seeking individual, who lacks a sense of responsibility, has little inclination for reflection, and no desire to dominate. He is a jolly fellow, prized for his optimism and jokes, his love for food, and his capacity for creating enjoyment. We recognize easily the *Calcarea carbonica* person who has gotten stuck in his individuation. These people often live in a world devoid of all imagination, entirely depending upon their sense perception. For them, the future is just a repetition of the past. The more sensation predominates, the more the suppressed intuition function forms projections: insane jealousy if the object is a sexual one. Such primitive erotomania and jealousy is seen in *Hyoscyamus* and *Apis*, both crude pleasure seekers and intensely possessive characters.

A dulling of sensation occurs when another function (feeling, thinking, or intuition) is predominant. For instance, the **introverted** sensation-thinking type is like a photographic plate—everything to which it is exposed leaves a mark on it. One of the biggest drawbacks in this type is his lack of spontaneity; he remains aloof and indifferent. This sensation-thinking type is definitely oriented to the facts and sees everything as rather static, so confusion easily sets in when something he considered to be so genuine turns out to be a trivial matter. The sensation type can adapt automatically to a situation or a person, out of laziness or not wanting to offend the other party. **Introverted**-sensation types might linger in such a blissful state but will make an awkward, difficult, and tedious partner in a marriage.

Prototype of introvert-sensation type: *Graphites!* (Did Jung have some *Graphites* in him?) Emma Jung alluded to this sensation-thinking type (see stocky build of Jung in pictures).

According to Jung the sensation type refers to a personality that has a little chip (or a big one) on his shoulder. In the eyes of the sensation type, others are inferior, which immediately evokes the pictures of *Platina*, *Palladium*, and even *Staphysagria* (delusion, *humility and lowness of others, while he is great*). Of course, other delusions express the same: *he is great; he is tall; does not belong to her family;* and *had grown tall while walking* (*Palladium*). The sensation type also belongs to the *Carbon* group. For more information, see *Hahnemann Revisited*, Chapter 8, page 142.

Chapter 12: The Active Miasmatic State

Question 10: What Is the Patient's Active Miasmatic State?

Chronic Diseases: The Importance of Miasmatic Prescribing

Already in Questions 3 and 5 we alluded to the importance of recognizing the active miasmatic state of the patient. Knowing the active miasmatic state helps the homeopath, at the end of his investigation, to narrow down his list of possible remedies. In order to have a deep-working action on the pathology of the patient, the selected remedy must cover the active miasm of the layer being treated. If the homeopath is not clear on the active miasmatic state, he risks choosing a very superficial remedy or even a wrong remedy, which can never eradicate the entire disease. This is one of the main reasons why a homeopath might initially have "success" with a patient, but then find no further progress or even a worsening of the natural disease, at best, palliation, but not a step towards cure. What Hahnemann wrote in 1828 in *Chronic Diseases* is still relevant today:

CD What was the reason of the thousands of unsuccessful endeavors to heal the other diseases of a chronic nature so that lasting health might result? Might this be caused, perhaps, by the still too small number of Homeopathic remedial means that have so far been proved as to their pure action? The followers of Homeopathy have hitherto thus consoled themselves; but this excuse, or so-called consolation, never satisfied the founder of Homeopathy—particularly because even the new additions of proved valuable medicines, increasing from year to year, have not advanced the healing of chronic (non-venereal) diseases by a single step, while acute diseases (unless these, at their commencement, threaten unavoidable death) are not only passably removed, by means of correct application of Homeopathic remedies, but with the assistance of the never-resting, preservative vital force in our organism, find a speedy and complete cure.

Why, then, cannot the vital force, efficiently affected through Homeopathic medicine, produce any true and lasting recovery in these chronic maladies even with the aid of the Homeopathic remedies which best cover their present symptoms; while this same force which is created for the restoration of our organism is nevertheless so indefatigably and successfully active in completing the recovery even in severe acute diseases? What is there to prevent this?

The answer to this question, which is so natural, inevitably led me to the discovery of the nature of these chronic diseases (1997, Vol. 1, pp. 4-5).

—

Hahnemann's every word is to be given great thought. He talks about the necessity of approaching *chronic*, not acute diseases with a miasmatic analysis. When Hahnemann started his work on the chronic miasms in 1816, it was because he was frustrated by the lack of success he had had in curing chronic diseases. If even Hahnemann had those problems, the present-day homeopath is confronted with many more suppressions of chronic diseases: the necessity of selecting the simillimum based on the miasmatic nature of the disease is mandated more than ever. Otherwise, the homeopath is only practicing "in the dark," and only by pure chance is he so fortunate as to find the simillimum.

Therefore, after answering the question—**What is the active miasmatic state of my patient?**—be sure the active miasm fits your chosen simillimum. For example, if the active miasmatic state of the patient is luetic (syphilitic), then the selected remedy should be a strongly anti-syphilitic one. Currently, we have no accurate books that describe the miasmatic make-up of each remedy. It is your responsibility to match the proving symptoms of your simillimum to the different miasms they express. This certainly is not an easy task for anyone, but reading *Hahnemann Revisited* and Chapter 15 in this book will greatly help you make this determination.

Check and Treat Latent Miasms and Family Miasms

It is also important to pay attention to *latent* miasmatic symptoms. For instance, consider recurrent nosebleeds. The patient, and sometimes even the homeopath, might think it is not important to treat this expression and so might not take it into account when selecting the simillimum. However, if one knows that this expression is a latent symptom of the psoric miasm, it pays to check whether other symptoms perceived in the patient belong to the psoric miasm. This latent symptom is like a dark warrior, hiding behind a closed door, ready to attack when weakness is perceived. Therefore, the homeopath must view this as a preliminary warning for an outbreak of a miasm and must treat even the latent miasmatic symptom before it bursts out in full force. This is truly preventive medicine. Note that nosebleeds are not some form of detoxification but rather an expression of Aphorisms 201 and 202, where Hahnemann tells us that the body's natural defense system or Vital Force (VF) continually pushes an internal disease to the surface so we can be alerted to its presence. Here again it is vital for the homeopath to understand miasmatic theory!

Make sure to check carefully the miasms in the family history. Pay attention to how there is often a cross-over between the sexes: for the male, I look at the mother's personal history; for the female at the father's history. Of course, the miasmatic background is often so strong on both sides that it would be a sheer miracle if the children escaped the taint of the family miasms. Also, consider that one partner may "catch" or obtain a miasm from the other, for example, when sudden pathology (such as vaginal yeast infections) develops upon marriage or sexual intercourse. This is not a case of "being allergic to your spouse" as allopathy often tries to explain. Both partners must be homeopathically treated or the ping-pong effect will keep the miasm alive.

Do not assume that two miasms are active at the same time. If two or more miasms are active that would indicate the cancer miasm! You might see symptoms of two different miasms in the history intake, but the homeopath must build a careful *timeline* in order to see what the most recent disease expressions are and to which miasm they belong. This often confirms, as Hahnemann preached in *Chronic Diseases*, that, "the stronger miasm will put the weaker in latency and that after curing the stronger one, the weaker will appear." In *Chronic Diseases*, Hahnemann writes:

> **CD** I have, in my practice, found only two cases of the threefold complication of the chronic miasms, the figwart disease with the venereal chancre miasm and at the same time a developed psora, and these cases were cured according to the same method; i.e., the psora was treated first, then the one of the other two chronic miasmata, the symptoms of which were at the time the most prominent, and then the last one The remaining psoric symptoms had then still to be combated with suitable remedies, and then lastly what there yet remained of sycosis or syphilis, by means of the remedies given above (1997, p. 95).

This paragraph does *not* indicate, as some homeopaths claim, that "Hahnemann alternated remedies." He tells us to use a new, different remedy only when *new symptoms* belonging to the next active miasmatic layer show up, *not* before they are indicated.

The timeline, therefore, needs to be compiled with the correct dates: if cysts, shingles, influenza, herpes, and myomata are all part of the latest history of the patient, and although she mentions having suffered earlier from eczema, vertigo, and tinnitus, we see clearly that, at present, the sycotic miasm has suspended the psoric one!

Question 11: In What Miasmatic State of the Selected Remedy Is the Patient? Psoric? Sycotic? Syphilitic?

Once the homeopath has determined the simillimum, it is important to note which miasmatic stage of the selected remedy is presented in the natural disease process. Each patient has different ways of compensating for their internal imbalance. And each remedy can address these compensations. Typically, at the onset of a disease state, the patient expresses positive compensations. It is the nature of the beast, so to speak, that the patient will try to do something positive in order to dissolve or support their core delusion. This refers to the psoric phase of the natural disease process, which stands for giving and/or receiving support! Each remedy has symptoms that correlate to each miasm: psoric, sycotic, and syphilitic. Disease compensations may start out being psoric, but over time they may advance to sycotic compensations and later syphilitic compensations, depending on the patient's miasmatic tendencies, life events, constitution, and other factors. For some remedies, for example the great syphilitic ones, *Mercurius, Aurum, Alumina, Kali iodatum*, etc., the psoric period can be very short-lived. But strong psoric characters, like *Arsenicum* and *Calcarea carbonica*, remain stubbornly on the positive compensation pathway. Look at the example of *Lachesis* in Chapter 7, the homeopath can always see an evolution according to the three great Hahnemannian miasms, going in their compensations from a support-seeking psoric state, to a frantic sycotic state (an exaggerated effort to obtain results), and ultimately, to the destructive syphilitic state where the patient gives up and withdraws.

Why Should We Try to Determine the Stage?

• First, it will tell the homeopath something about the actual dominant miasm of the patient and his compensations. The psoric person will do anything to remain as long as possible in the psoric phase and avoid the syphilitic one. His psoric compensations are numerous: stubbornness, looking for company, industriousness, conscientiousness, religion, music, etc. In this case, the chosen remedy should be outspokenly psoric. On the other hand, the syphilitic person quickly falls into a destructive cycle as he lacks sympathy, insight, remorse, and moral feeling.

• Second, if the patient shows mainly psoric expressions (compensations) of the simillimum and remains in this phase for a long time, the *prognosis*, and therefore healing time, is very favorable, no matter what the official diagnosis is! For instance, the miasmatic disease phase can show the homeopath the difference between a slowly developing multiple sclerosis (MS) case and a quickly progressing one. Where allopathy struggles to understand why some cases of MS evolve slowly but others rapidly, the homeopath knows that in the slow-moving cases the dominant miasm is psoric while in the fast-moving cases, sycosis has combined with this syphilitic illness. Another useful piece of information!

• Third, this tells you what *kind of patient* you are dealing with. The psoric person will most likely follow your instructions, be cooperative, and ask for close supervision. But he will be locked into small details (much ado about nothing) and will often fail to register important emotional changes (*Calcarea carbonica, Arsenicum*). The syphilitic patient will most likely disregard your advice, refuse to take the remedy as he tells you that "nothing will help," or cancel the homeopathic remedy's action with destructive behavior (e.g., drugs, alcohol, etc.). The sycotic patient will double the dose of his medicine, just because he "loves the juice and the zip" it gives his body. "Wow, these are great drugs," he says. The sycotic type may be very suspicious of your remedy, having the *delusion that the medicine is poison.* Mixed miasmatic states have different reactions. *Carcinosin* will be meticulous and sensitive to each reaction of his body. The tubercular patient will often become quickly disenchanted and either abandon homeopathic treatment or combine his therapy with the "latest miracle" supplements and modalities.

• Fourth, the homeopath gets to know each remedy in its full picture, not *only in its end-stage* or syphilitic stage—what is usually taught in schools and books!

• Last but not least, the homeopath can see that the case is moving according to Hering's Set of Observations when he sees the sycotic phase of the remedy picture shifting to the psoric phase (see Chap. 16).

Miasms: It's All About the Terrain!

Even with my advanced students, I observe the mistaken presumption that a miasm is caused by a virus, a bacteria, a tick bite, etc. It is not the germ; it's the terrain that is all-important! Why doesn't everyone develop Lyme disease when bitten by a tick? In all clinically positive Lyme patients, the tick bite from a tick carrying the bacteria that causes Lyme disease was the proverbial straw that broke the camel's back. But before the person could acquire this disease, they must have a prior history of great stress (emotional, physical, or mental). These patients, each in their own words, often express how they have nothing left to fight with.

The patient's miasmatic soil and constitution dictate how they express their unique symptoms and the common, albeit variable, symptoms of Lyme disease. *The tick bite does nothing unless the terrain is weakened and receptive!* The homeopath must not be scared by microbes, yeast, etc., or by the name of the disease. A microbe does *not create* any miasm: its reaction depends on the strength of the VF and on the miasmatic genetic background of the patient or as Jung calls it, the fixed and mandated (not chosen) predisposed response pattern.

So now we see the big difference between the allopath's approach and homeopath's approach to infection. Allopaths kill off microorganisms by using drugs in physiological doses. Unfortunately, this leads to drug-resistant microorganisms, especially after repeated drug use. Homeopathic remedies stimulate the natural defensive mechanism, which becomes stronger than the disease force, thereby killing these microorganisms indirectly through the creation of inhospitable terrain for their survival and multiplication. Homeopathic remedies never create resistant microorganisms, and, moreover, the natural defense mechanism (VF, Qi, immune system) becomes stronger due to the gentle, yet powerful, action of the remedies.

Chapter 13: Intrauterine Questions for Cases of Challenged Children

The Latest Allopathic Findings

In my local newspaper, *The Santa Fe New Mexican*, August 24, 2005, I read an article titled, *Researchers: Fetuses feel no pain until final months*. The report appeared in that month's issue of the *Journal of the American Medical Association* and the study was done by researchers at the University of California, San Francisco. It all had to do with the abortion issue, of course, and affirmed that, "while brain structures involved in feeling pain begin forming much earlier than the seventh month of pregnancy, research indicates they likely do not function." To be fair, not every fetal-pain researcher agreed with these findings.

I do not need such a study because I see how the fetus is influenced from *day one* of its existence by psychic pain endured by the mother. Homeopaths frequently see examples of challenged children whose mother suffered from an emotional stress (feeling forsaken, grief, deception, hearing bad news, etc.). This book cites several examples. Homeopaths can attest to this psychological "infection," and if psychological pain transferred from the mother can be felt, so can physical pain.

Obtaining Information About the Pregnancy: A Hornet's Nest!

If the homeopath thinks that obtaining information from his patient regarding her most intimate history may be difficult, he has not faced yet the hurdles of obtaining input from the mother regarding emotional traumas while she was pregnant and how these events most likely caused the symptoms affecting her challenged child. The reasons for this are clear.

First, the mother of a challenged child already feels enough guilt and sorrow that her child has a problem, often sexual or criminal in nature, or has behavior problems at school and at home. Trying to pinpoint a clear **intrauterine** causality, possibly linked to the mother's thoughts or actions, is enough to push the evidence into the unconscious.

Secondly, and often a worse scenario, is that the mother probably has to draw other people into the picture, often close family, her parents or the father, to explain the circumstances of the trauma. Family members often play a role in instigating the "trauma," which is often an unconscious action on their part. The mother may not be inclined to discuss such events: "Let's let sleeping dogs lie!"

But, before pointing an accusing finger at anyone (which the homeopath should always avoid doing, in any event), he had better consider the repercussions that even the slightest allusion to such a trauma may have! This might be the last time he sees his patient!

Third and foremost, in answering, "How was your pregnancy," the mother will most likely only concentrate on the physical aspect of her pregnancy, unless she was seriously depressed, in a serious accident, or involved in a more blatant trauma. If no physical problems such as nausea, threatened miscarriage, bleeding, mal-position of the fetus, etc. were present, she will say everything was OK! The most important triggers, the mental/emotional ones, which may explain the unfortunate situation of a challenged child, can remain unclear and uninvestigated not only by allopaths, but also by homeopaths.

It remains a mystery why allopaths, even in the 21st century, are so far removed from seeing a link between the mother's emotions and the repercussions on the fetus, something confirmed for a long time by Traditional Chinese Medicine (TCM) and even more so by homeopathy. In *The Foundations of Chinese Medicine*, Giovanni Maciocia and Churchill Livingstone note in their chapter on "Causes of Disease" that: "A severe shock to the mother during pregnancy will affect the constitution of the baby, particularly the Heart. This is often manifested with a bluish tinge on the forehead and on the chin" (1989, p. 135). However, nothing more is said in TCM about this very important issue of intrauterine trauma. Homeopathy, with its clear patterns of proven remedies, can pin-point the trauma and deliver therapeutic measures better than any other modality.

My guess is that allopathy has difficulty confirming such a link because it tends to confirm its diagnoses with blood tests, X-rays, and other technical findings. Obviously, such measures will not gauge the fetus' emotions. I bet they would like to do PET scans of the brains of pregnant moms to see if maternal emotions change the fetal brain picture, but none has yet been taken. And what if allopathy finds irregularities on such scans? Will that result in a therapeutic intervention? I would not be surprised if allopathy were to start giving tranquilizers and anti-depressants to the pregnant mother.

Because the gynecologist and pediatrician never ask such "touchy" questions to see if there might have been transference of emotions from the mother to the fetus, mothers never even think about it when the physician or homeopath asks them, "How was your pregnancy?" "Just fine," they will say. And unfortunately, too many homeopaths will take such an answer at face value, missing one of the most important pieces of the child's simillimum: the true Never Well Since (NWS) event or trigger. If the homeopath wants to find the simillimum, he needs to go to the place of the trauma. Any good crime detective will go to the scene of the crime to find out what is "unusual, peculiar, and outstanding," conducting an "Aphorism 153" investigation!

One word of caution to the homeopath: be very diplomatic with the patient; don't be blunt, cold, or intrusive when you ask these questions. The patient has probably never been asked such questions, so don't continue immediately with another question after you finish one: give the mom time to think it over. No cross examinations! Watch her body language, telltale indicators such as hesitations, sudden tears, or Freudian slips can provide you with information regarding the trigger. If the homeopath observes such behavior (proof that he has touched upon a sensitive issue), she should tell the mother gently that this information is very important in resolving her child's illness! No mother will refuse such a request! It might be painful; it might be buried deep inside; she may even have thought all along that it might have affected her baby. In any event, all of this can be a shock once it is revealed! Don't act like a prosecutor out on a vendetta! Here more than ever, the homeopath must mimic the dominant function of the patient's consciousness (see Ch. 10).

The following questions are important because they are often linked to "ailments from," which in turn belong to important remedies that fit the picture of the challenged child (ADD, ADHD, ASD or Autism Spectrum Disorder, OCD, etc.).

INTRAUTERINE QUESTIONS

1. Was the pregnancy planned? First reaction?
2. Was the pregnancy desired by your partner and family?
3. Any estrangement or separation from your partner, family or friends?
4. Any conflicts with your partner and/or family?
5. Any deaths or bad news during pregnancy?
6. Mental and/or physical overwork?
7. Any emotional events?
8. Any change in family dynamics?
9. Cravings and/or aversions? Other stressors? How was birthing process?
10. Physical condition and age of parents at conception?

---

1. Was the pregnancy planned? Was it the right moment? What was your (the mom's) first reaction when you heard that you were pregnant?

The first person in line to alter the psychology of the pregnancy's mental/ emotional state is the mother. The first reaction triggers initial changes, since she is the first to hear the news that she is pregnant or at least correctly assumes she is when she feels the changes in her body. Pregnancies often come as a surprise, so the very first reaction might be, "Oh, not right now! I am just not ready for this because …" School, job, moving, relationship not going well, being physically and emotionally overwhelmed, and probably 100 other reasons may worry the perspective mother. I have even heard remarks like, "My pregnancy with her was the reason my career never got off the ground."

I have been told, "I got pregnant on the pill (yes, it can happen!), and I was not sure I wanted the baby. I did not like the changes in my body, and I was very doubtful I could be a good mother since I had a history of bad temper." It is interesting to see that this particular "mental/emotional rejection" of the fetus was followed by the body's attempt to physically reject the fetus. In her last three weeks of pregnancy, she was hospitalized with toxemia (BP 220/190), and the baby came out in a big gush of green water. The mother went on, "The placenta had died and had not been nurturing him for weeks. He was five pounds at birth. He refused the nipple and cried constantly, so I went into a total state of postpartum depression in which I was afraid I would hurt him (indication for *Sepia*!!)."

Some women do not like to be pregnant in the first place. Some do not like to become "fat" as they think it makes them ugly. Others are exhausted throughout the pregnancy. I had a patient who said she "resented being tied down in bed for hyperemesis gravidarum, a threatening miscarriage, and the feeling of being trapped" (as she was unable to go anywhere). Another pregnant mom felt that her unborn child was "like an alien, sucking all the energy out of me." The brunt of these emotions will be carried over to the unborn fetus.

The thought, "I can't be pregnant right now" means outright **rejection** of the fetus' first days of life, an unconscious refusal to bond with the fetus. It might even get worse when the pregnant mom is plagued by strong nausea and vomiting (hyperemesis gravidarum), which might also evoke negative feelings towards the unborn baby. The homeopath should therefore ask the first emotional reaction of the mom. Was it joy, anger, frustration, shock—or maybe sadness because you always wanted to be pregnant to give your parents a grandchild, but now they are deceased? Now this happy news can accentuate buried grief and cause it to resurface, making the mother long for what *might* have been: happy moments with her parents (*homesickness*). Sadness might also overshadow the happy news because the relationship with the husband is not right or the mother-to-be is unmarried.

Here is another story: the mother was disappointed when she was given the "bad news" that her baby was a boy, because she wanted a girl. To make things worse, she was given the additional bad news that her unborn son "might" have spina bifida, a congenital spinal defect. For some time she was horrified, hysterical, crying non-stop. She might have to abort the child and that conflicted with her religious beliefs. The results came back negative a week later, and it turned out to be false alarm. But the damage was done. Her child is now full of fears, greatly affected when he sees children with cancer on TV, fears people will hurt him, and exhibits great fears of the dark, thunderstorms, etc. The foundation for his temperament and behavior was laid down **intrauterine** through the mother's unfortunate desire for a girl, and by her anticipation fears, which created a mistuned constitution.

Reality is often more bizarre and complicated than anything a homeopath could invent. One of my patients was known as "the good one" in her family. She was going to nursing school and was busy. She wasn't married but was dating a man who was not supposed to be able to produce children (only an irreversible vasectomy can guarantee this!) When she learned she was pregnant, it was a great shock (*hearing bad news*). Then she felt embarrassed: "I am the good one in the family. I'm not married and here I am, pregnant! What will people say about me when they find out?"

She felt her family would be disappointed with her and cried when she first heard the news. She seemed to get over it all in a relatively short period of time, became excited, and started putting things in order: planning a wedding, looking for future baby sitters, finishing nursing school, etc. During the process, she often felt frustration towards her future husband as she liked things to be a certain way. She said she did not like to express negative emotions so she kept most of them in. Towards the end of the pregnancy, there was much emotional excitement and anticipation, followed by the big let-down when her baby was born. She then suffered from postpartum depression while feeding the baby, which transferred many negative emotions to the baby!

Most people fail to understand that even if the emotion is only present for a few days, even hours, the impact on the fetus can be great. This is easily seen in cases where there are two or more children in the family and only one is challenged. The homeopath should immediately investigate these pregnancies, looking for an emotional trigger where the child was born challenged! Compare the different pregnancies and ask the mom, "What do you think was different in the pregnancy that resulted in this challenged child?" The reasons are often unimaginable, as evidenced by the examples in this book.

2. Was the pregnancy desired by your partner and/or family?

Emotional trauma may also be traced back to the immediate family: husband, parents from both sides, even the extended family and close friends! The expectant mother is extremely sensitive to negative comments and criticism from others, especially from those who are supposed to be a source of support, sharing in her joy! Don't underestimate the expectant mother's reactions. The man in her life is often not ready to be a father (or be a father again!) "I wanted to enjoy our freedom and travel a little first." "We cannot afford a second child." "One child is enough for us." "I am not ready to get married and settle down." All this comes across as rejection (*forsaken*), bad news, even a betrayal to the expectant mom (*ailments from disappointed love*)! If the husband is present at the first consultation, you might want to send him out while you ask this question.

During the pregnancy, the husband may resent receiving less attention and may withdraw from his wife. Grandparents may not be pleased about another grand-child, and may not be enthusiastic even though it's the first pregnancy for this woman. Or the family might say, "There is no way you can take care of this baby, you're still a child yourself!" Of course, some expectant, unwed mothers are very young and often don't get support or an enthusiastic response from the parents or boyfriend. Even if the family becomes excited, the damage is done. In such cases, mothers often forget and will say, "Of course my husband and parents were happy when they knew I was pregnant!"

3. Any estrangement or separation from your partner, family, or friends during the pregnancy? Was your partner mostly at home or did he travel for work?

Ask these questions to probe for states of *fright and abandonment*, two of the most frequent and important NWS (ailments from) in a challenged child. Pregnancy, especially first-time pregnancy, is often a period of increased anxiety. Kent compares the primigravida (first-time pregnant patient) to a nervous race horse; *Aconite* is a remedy often needed for the fearful expectant mom. She may fear that something will go wrong; that the delivery will be extremely painful; that she might die; that she will not have enough food for the baby; that she did something during the pregnancy which might harm the baby, etc. This frame of mind often leads to miscarriages for which *Aconite* is **the** indicated remedy.

What if the patient already has one challenged child and now she is pregnant for the second time? There will surely be anguish and anticipation anxiety, carried over to the unborn fetus. It is evident that for many women pregnancy represents a period of increased emotional and physical need for support. Where beforehand these women seemed strong, even independent, pregnancy demands a close support group—husband, family and friends, in that order. Even reduced contact with friends during pregnancy might be felt as betrayal or as abandonment. Even when the work situation of the husband has not changed, the "neediness" of the pregnant mother increases, a natural reaction, not pathology!

All this gets worse if the husband suddenly has to travel for his work and is perhaps even away for weeks on end. Even if this was something she was used to before the pregnancy, now it's a different ballgame. "I want my husband close to home … just in case something happens." This situation often puts the mother into an *Argentum nitricum* state: "What if I can't reach my husband?" "What if this or that happens?" "What if I start bleeding or my contractions begin?" More often than not, this certainly may be the case for the more fearful carbon people (*Kali carbonicum, Calcarea carbonica*), *Arsenicum*, and related remedies (*Kali arsenicum, Calcarea arsenica*) and for the sensitive and phobic *Phosphorus*, a natural bleeder, which often creates situations of early bleeding. Where normally the husband's absence never evoked an particular feeling, now it is translated as "abandonment!" "You were not there for me when I needed you," is the battle cry, and the trauma has occurred. Don't be surprised to find "primitive," hysterical emotions in otherwise very intelligent people during pregnancy.

It is quite possible that pregnancy changes the usual dominant function of conscious. For example, the thinking person (especially *Lachesis* and *China*, which are passionate and paranoid remedies with delusions of persecution) may turn into an archaic, primitive feeling-type person, evoking all kinds of emotions, even jealousy and suspicion. The homeopath can see how, during pregnancy, *Lachesis* takes on many *Natrum muriaticum* aspects: taciturn, irritable, withdrawn, etc. This easily leads to an estrangement from the husband—or the expectant mother perceives estrangement where there is none. "Of course he does not want me any more; I am ugly and fat. He's probably looking for another wife" (delusions: *is forsaken and is unfortunate* [China]; *he is sent to the mental asylum*; [Lachesis]; *or a lover is behind the stove* [Hyoscyamus]). The homeopath must remember that pregnancy can be a period where miasmatic states wake up, for example, awakening the sycotic miasm might mean an early miscarriage or a possible resurgence of jealousy and suspicion.

Family members, especially, can do unintended damage. Now that the expectant mother has such happy news, she may hope for reunion and closeness with her parents after a long estrangement, but may receive a cold or even indifferent response. I have even heard parents commenting to their pregnant daughter who needed urgent, possibly life-saving intervention that "everything is in God's hands now; there is no need for us to come." Resulting emotions can include feelings of being forsaken, of unrequited love, being treated rudely, anger, disbelief, grief, etc. It all depends on how the expectant mother reacts to such comments. Don't just guess, ask the patient how she felt! What is certain: the unborn fetus has been subjected to the mother's emotions!

4. Did you have any conflicts with your partner and/or family?

Incidents of discord are easily forgotten, especially if afterwards everything was fine. "Did you experience periods of tension between you and your husband and/or family?" *Ailments from discord between chief and subordinates* is a frequent causality, which provokes all kinds of emotions in the expectant mother and fetus. Make sure you get to the bottom of the issue and ask the mother, "How did you react to this discord? How did you feel? What was your dominant emotion in regard to this event? How long did the feeling last? Did the incident leave a permanent scar? Do you still think about this (*sad thoughts, persistent*)?" As one mother expressed it: "My anger towards my husband lasted longer than my entire pregnancy!"

5. Did anyone close to you die or did you receive any bad news during your pregnancy?

Hearing bad news is always a shock to the system, and its effects should not be underestimated. Pregnancy puts a woman into a very sensitive or receptive state, so the trauma is always felt more strongly. How the patient reacted to the bad news will tell you much about the possible remedy and the active miasmatic state of the mom and the fetus. "I could not move upon hearing the news, I felt paralyzed (*Gelsemium*)." Or, "I sobbed all day long" (*Ignatia*). Or, "I totally fell apart and became indecisive and obsessed with details" (*Silica*). Or, "I felt the need to close myself up in my home and phone all my friends" (*Calcarea carbonica*).

All these important remedies can be used for the different ways people respond to hearing bad news. Unfortunately, emotional trauma can also lead to *physically* challenged children. I had a case of a five-year-old child whose father had died in a car accident while mom was pregnant. This child had impeded speech, was late talking, and underwent no fewer than three unsuccessful operations. Mom's indicated grief remedy was also the remedy that corrected the child's speech. For example, if a sensitive, justice-oriented person like *Causticum*, *Phosphorus*, *Aurum*, or *Lachesis* hears bad news related to a world event, often war crimes, she can easily transfer her emotions onto the fetus.

Hearing bad news can affect the present pregnancy and even the *next one*. I had the tragic example of a friend who went to prison unjustly for eight days. During this ordeal, his wife was pregnant for the second time and immediately miscarried. When she got pregnant again months later, she was still in such a state of neediness, fright, and grief that this second child was born mentally challenged, where the first born child was totally normal.

6. Did you experience physical and/or mental overwork?

Be sure to ask, "Did you continue working? How long did you work? Did your work situation change during the pregnancy (more responsibility or more tasks than usual)? Did you have to stop working; what was your reaction to this? Were you feeling overwhelmed by what you already needed to do?" This is especially true if the mother has other children. Be sure to ask how many years apart the children are. "How were your most recent pregnancies/deliveries? Did you experience morning sickness, postpartum depression, or other illnesses?"

We must pay special attention to ailments from mental overload (*ailments from mental exertion* [*Nux vomica*, 4]; *mental work fatigues* [*Nux vomica*, 2]; or *mental work is impossible* [*Nux vomica*, 2]). Because *Nux vomica* is the acute complement of *Sepia*, we know that there is a danger for miscarriage (months 5 to 7) and of course postpartum depression. Consider other black-type remedies that are aggravated by mental exertion: *Argentum nitricum*, *Lachesis*, *Lycopodium*, *Natrum carbonicum*, *Natrum muriaticum*, *Staphysagria*, and *Tuberculinum*; any of these remedies may be intimately connected with the birth of a challenged child.

7. Did you have any frequently occurring emotional events like: situations at work or home that triggered indignation; frights; jealousy; grief; deception; financial strain?

Inquire about these strong emotions, especially situations of fright, which are a big source of NWS events for many different remedies and are usually not asked about. "Did you experience any frightening events (murder, accident, suicide, robbery, fire, something going wrong in the pregnancy, etc.)?" Grief, deception, and indignation usually stick in the patient's mind. You have only to think of "fright" remedies like *Stramonium*, *Hyoscyamus*, *Opium*, *Gelsemium*, *Lycopodium*, and *Pulsatilla* to realize that they all play a role in many autistic children. This is also the moment dormant or latent miasms will become active, triggered by the frightening event.

8. Any change in the family dynamics? Did you have to pay more attention to those living with you (mother, relative, other children)?

Make sure to ask if the family dynamic changed during the pregnancy because this can add extra stress on the expectant mother. It could be a stepchild or mother or mother-in-law moving in. Perhaps another child in the family became very sick, demanding more of the mother's attention. Perhaps the step-child came on a two-month vacation at the end of a most stressful pregnancy. Another example from my practice is that the husband was diagnosed with cancer before his wife became pregnant but both decided that they had always wanted to be parents and went ahead with the attempt at pregnancy. However, the soon-to-be mother initially reacted to her husband's diagnosis with terror, which shocked her to the core of her being. This incident in itself decreases the Essence of this patient, setting the stage for a problematic child (see Question 10). Most of that expectant mother's pregnancy would then have to be geared towards her husband's treatments, possibly causing feelings of abandonment and emotional excitement (stress). This is of course also a change in the family dynamic because the husband would become a lot more dependent on his wife.

9. Did you have any food cravings or aversions? Alcohol intake? Smoking habits? How was the birthing process? What was the baby's Apgar score? Any emotional stresses during breast feeding?

Cravings and aversions are important because they signal the miasm carried over from the husband to the expectant mother. Pica gravidarum (cravings in pregnancy) are an important piece of information for the homeopath on which he needs to act immediately to ensure the good health of the mother and future child! There is no doubt that every pregnant woman should have homeopathic treatment, if possible before getting pregnant!

The birthing process is equally important. We are especially concerned about head trauma (forceps, suction, prolonged duration of labor), which might require a remedy like *Helleborus*, *Thuja*, or *Cicuta*, depending on the picture. Certainly, such sycotic/syphilitic remedies are a solution for ADD and ASD children. Emotional trauma can also occur during delivery. One of my patients described it succinctly: "Upon our arrival in the hospital, my husband fainted. All the nurses were preoccupied with him as I was struggling with my labor pains. My husband always seems to attract the interest of women (a pang of jealousy?). I felt very angry and abandoned at this moment, yes even insulted."

The result was a restless, very needy, and often angry child, labeled, of course ADHD, but the case was a *Tarentula* child.

Even if everything was OK during pregnancy and delivery, the child continues to be influenced by emotional traumas during the **breastfeeding** period. *Ignatia* shows such close association in its provings, *infantile colic after taking breast of mother, who suffers from grief* (Hering). It's like feeding grief to the baby! So the homeopath must take into account the mother's mental/emotional state during breast feeding. Another example is epilepsy in a child when the mother had a fright during the nursing period: *The child became epileptic in consequence of mother having a fright or fit of anger during nursing period*, a *Bufo* proving symptom.

10. What was your physical condition and age at the time of conception? Your partner's condition and age?

I am interested in what allopathy has to say about this issue. The phrase "my biological clock is ticking" used to refer only to females, but now there is evidence that men are also ticking off some of their healthy children," says Jay Schinfeld, a fertility specialist at Abrington Reproductive Medicine. The latest findings suggest that older fathers are more likely to have children with autism. The odds of fathering an autistic child are about 6 in 1,000 for men under 20. When a man reaches 50 (way beyond what TCM favors as reproductive age), those odds shoot up to about 52 in 1,000. "The optimal time for a man to father a healthy child is the same as for a woman—25 or so," says Dolores Malaspina, a professor of psychiatry at New York University and co-author of the study.

This same physician also conducted a study showing a connection between paternal age and schizophrenia. She found children born to fathers over 50 carried about three times the risk of developing schizophrenia of those born to fathers in their 20s.

While these same authors remain clueless about the reason behind these statistics (except for looking at the age statistics which do not provide a reason), the seasoned homeopath knows that this has everything to do with evolution from the psoric miasm to the sycotic or syphilitic miasm, which unfortunately appear at a younger and younger age in present-day society. Schizophrenia and most ASD cases are syphilitic expressions and in these instances, the homeopath will **always** be able to find the presence of the syphilitic miasm in the patient's family history, or what some scientists refer to as "spelling errors in the DNA."

These eminent specialists could learn something from TCM because the scientists' findings do not correspond with TCM's **findings**. In TCM, the **Water element (Kidney) stores Essence, which governs birth, growth, reproduction, and development.** This Essence received from the parents and partly replenished by the Qi extracted from food determines our basic constitution, strength, and vitality (i.e., our predominant miasm). The inherited constitution will depend on the strength and quality of the parent's Essence in general and at the time of conception in particular. If the parent's Essence is weak, the child's "Kidney" will be weak. This may manifest through poor bone development, mental retardation, pigeon chest, loose teeth, spina bifida, etc. In these expressions, we primarily see the manifestation of the syphilitic miasm.

The Kidney Essence is also the material foundation for the manufacturing of sperm in men and ova in women. Nowadays we see more and more infertility due to production of abnormal sperm and/or absence of sperm. In such cases, the Essence inherited from the parents is no doubt influenced by the syphilitic miasm! Abnormal sperm will respond rather well to homeopathy; absence of sperm would be more problematic. So, insufficient Essence may be the cause of infertility, impotence, and underdevelopment in children (physical or mental), retarded growth, and premature senility.

It goes without saying that, in looking at these factors, one of the most important aspects in the parents' supplying the child with a good Essence is their **age**. Since Kidney Essence declines with age, if the parents conceive when they are too old, their child's constitution might suffer. For TCM, the ideal age for a woman to conceive is between 28 and 35, for men, the ideal age is between 32 and 40 (note how different these figures are from those quoted by the allopathic fertility specialists!) The homeopath needs to think about this as women become pregnant via fertility drugs at an older age. Similarly, if the parents are in a state of **exhaustion** at the time of conception, this may also cause a hereditary weakness of their child. This may explain the sometimes striking difference in physical appearance and personality amongst siblings.

An example of a tennis friend of mine showed this clearly. He has three children, the youngest being 6 years old, the older ones 9 and 11. He told me that his youngest son broke his femur in a simple fall, that he had already broken his humerus at age one, and that he also suffered from a hearing defect. These are all expressions of a deficient Kidney Essence. In fact, I did not have to ask if this was the youngest child. The two older children did not suffer at all from these problems so the age of parents at conception (father was 47; mother was 43) was past the ideal moment to conceive a child. In addition, the mother was in a *Sepia* state, which contributed to these "syphilitic" defects in the youngest child!

Having looked at all these questions, I marvel at the fact that there is even one healthy baby born into this world!

PART 2: ADVANCED MANAGEMENT

The Great Homeopathic Debate

From homeopathy's early years till now, the debate between low and high potency prescribers rages on. Not one topic creates more confusion and causes more feathers to fly, yet it is essential for homeopaths to come to a sensible consensus. Tempers flare and everyone claims success with their potency selection. While I have no doubt that both camps, the low and high potency prescribers, are correct to some extent, there must be a middle way, one that originates from reasoning, not passion. I want to emphasize that I'm talking about the "potency" (strength) of the remedy, not the "dose" (amount administered). I am continually surprised that homeopaths worldwide confuse these terms, whereas eminent homeopaths from Hahnemann to H.R. Roberts have made a clear distinction between the two concepts. The great culprit here was James Tyler Kent who stated that the dose made no difference. Many present-day homeopaths follow his lead, creating similar aggravations (and dissimilar ones) that turn patients away from homeopathy, never to return. In this chapter, I discuss not only potency selection, but also the dosing of the remedy. Homeopaths who claim that it does not matter whether you give three pellets or 10, three drops or a whole 4-oz. cup (and they are legion), must in my opinion be asleep at their job, since experience clearly shows that this does matter. May all homeopaths test the contents in this chapter for themselves! I am open to further discussion if they see things differently after trying what I suggest.

The Puzzling Reality in the Practice

Homeopaths see so many examples in practice that puzzle them: one person will react beautifully to a low potency, while another responds only to high potencies. One reacts to the C scale and not to LM potencies, while another patient appears to need LMs. No wonder homeopaths find it difficult to agree when they discuss potency selection. But there must be a plausible explanation for all this: some kind of middle road in the madness of determining the correct potencies. Here are some examples from actual practice that could create such confusion:

"I was using the 5th edition *Organon* split-dose method and giving *Phosphorus* 200C, repeated every two hours, for my daughter. It did nothing for her cold, which she'd had for three weeks. One single 10M dose and the next minute she was coughing up lots and lots of mucus, then she sat down and made jokes at dinner, then played with her brother and sister, which she had not done for four weeks. Ate voraciously and is still doing well. Cough has decreased from four times an hour with much expectoration to once every two to three hours" (i.e., *Phosphorus* 10M cured in one day, whereas 200C had no effect).

"I gave my aunt *Kali carbonicum* LM1 for spinal stenosis (she had all the keynotes of *Kali carbonicum*) with the following instructions: succuss the Remedy Stock Bottle (RSB) 2 times, dilute 1 tsp. of remedy from the RSB in 1 cup of water, and take 1 tsp. from the cup as needed (see *Achieving and Maintaining the Simillimum*, Chap. 4). I checked with her many times to see if she was taking the dose correctly. She said she was. When her bottle was finished, I found out that she had been drinking the whole cup each time she repeated a dose instead of taking 1 tsp., yet she had made splendid progress and is now 80 percent better."

"A 50-year-old lady reacted beautifully to 6C split-dose of *Natrum muriaticum*, bringing back old symptoms; improvement on all levels. After finishing the RSB of 6C, I changed to a 30C. She reported that she was continuing to do great, but that she "ran out of gas" a day and a half after each dose. Thinking she needed more "horsepower," I changed to LM1 with instructions to succuss the RSB 2 times, dilute 1 tsp. of remedy from the RSB in 1 cup of water, and take 1 tsp. from the cup. She had no response even when I increased the succussions." (On receiving a freshly made up bottle of LM1, the patient responded beautifully to the same dose! Were non-impregnated pellets used before? Most likely!)

"I seem to experience an aggravation for about four days after each dose of my remedy, then I do well for 14 days, but as soon as I repeat the dose, I go through the same cycle!" (This is a true hypersensitive and adjustment of dose/potency is necessary!)

In my practice I have many examples where three drops from the cup was too much and one drop did not do anything, but two drops of the remedy cured!

A Word About the Dose

When discussing potency selection, there is one golden rule for the practice: when using the C scale for chronic or acute cases, always choose the 5th edition split-dose method! With this method, the homeopath has many ways of adjusting the potency and dose (see *Achieving and Maintaining the Simillimum*, Chap. 4). The question I am posing in this section is, which potency does the homeopath select for diverse problems, *not the way* we administer it! Many homeopaths incorrectly assume that if the selection of the remedy is accurate, it will cure in iwhatever potency it is administered. They base this on the fact that Hahnemann "stated" in Aphorism 279 that the medicinal power can never be weaker than the disease power. But what did Hahnemann really say?

A 279 ... *the **dose*** [he says **dose**, not potency!] *of the highly potentized homeopathic remedy beginning the treatment of a significant (chronic) disease can, as a rule, not be made so small*

- *that it is not stronger than the natural disease,*
- *that it cannot at least partially overcome it,*
- *that it cannot at least partially extinguish it in the feelings of the vital principle,*
- *that it cannot start the process of cure.*

The exact definition of the simillimum is the correct remedy, potency, and dose for that case!

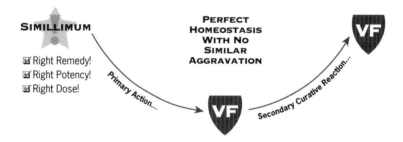

Let me stress once again: in this section of the book I am concentrating on the **potency** aspect, not the dose. For the latter, we adhere to Aphorism 279 and use the split-dose method described in the 5th edition of the *Organon* for C potencies or the LM method described in the 6th edition of the *Organon*.

Furthermore, concerning the dose of the remedy, Hahnemann states that:

A 280 One continues to give a medicine as long as it continues to benefit the patient and does not give rise to any new troublesome complaints [De Schepper notes: such as too many accessory symptoms or new symptoms], and one *gradually increases the dose* until the patient, *while feeling generally better*, begins at once to experience one or more of his old, original symptoms to a moderate degree. If the remedy has been modified each time by succussion (par. 247) and the very moderate doses have been gradually increased, this return of old symptoms indicates that cure is imminent, and that the vital principle has almost no more need to be affected by the similar medicinal disease in order to stop feeling the natural disease (par. 148), and that, now more free of the natural disease, it is beginning to suffer somewhat from the homeopathic medicinal disease, otherwise known as *homeopathic aggravation*.

The homeopath can clearly see how Hahnemann distinguishes between dose and potency! One more word of warning, in general, the homeopath can do a lot more harm with too large a dose and too frequent repetition than with too high a potency. If too high a potency is repeated at judicious intervals, then little harm will be done! Too large a dose and frequent repetition, even of the homeopathically selected remedy, will harm the patient to the point of making a case incurable. If too high a potency is repeated in the smallest **dose**, and repeated when the action of the previous dose has ceased, much less harm will be done. Regarding the dose, we can say, in general, that the closer the chosen remedy is to the simillimum, the less quantity of the drug is required. Roberts says:

> The greater the number of the characteristic symptoms of the disease that are found to correspond to the drug (similarity), the less the quantity and the higher the potency that can be used. ... In sickness susceptibility is markedly increased, as the avenues of diseased states are widely opened so that which would have an effect on health will be quickly grasped in disease. The resemblance of the group of symptoms is marked, therefore accordingly the very smallest possible dose will satisfy the susceptibility and therefore be curative (Roberts, 1986, pp. 121, 122).

In homeopathic terms, the patient's diseased part has a higher sensitivity to the simillimum, therefore the smallest dose will be curative!

In the above statement, Roberts is paraphrasing **Aphorism 277** of the *Organon*:

> **A 277** ... if the dose is appropriately small, a **well-dynamized** medicine becomes increasingly curative and almost miraculously helpful the more homeopathically it has been chosen, it follows that if a medicine is accurately homeopathic it must become increasingly beneficial as its dose approaches the ideal degree of smallness for gentle action (emphasis added).

I think the homeopath will do well to heed Hahnemann's words where he warns us about the dose and potency of the **simillimum**:

> **A 275** The correctness of a medicine for a given case of disease depends not only on its accurate homeopathic selection but also on the correct size (or rather **smallness**) of the dose. A medicine given in *too large dose*, **though completely homeopathic to the case** (emphasis added) and in itself of a beneficial nature, will still harm the patient by its quantity and unnecessarily strong action on the vital force, and through it, because the medicine is homeopathic, on precisely those parts of the organism which are most sensitive and have already been afflicted most by the natural disease.

Hahnemann explicitly talks about the large **dose** and reminds the homeopath that the diseased part of the patient is **highly sensitive to the remedy**; hence the smallest possible dose of the simillimum is required. This additional warning is for those who believe that "whenever they have the simillimum, the dose does not matter." Hahnemann says:

—

A 276 For this reason a medicine, although homeopathic to the case, does harm when it is given in **overdose**. In strong doses the more homeopathic the medicine and the higher its potency the more harm it does: indeed it is far more harmful than equally large doses of unhomeopathic medicine ... Excessively large **doses** of an accurately selected homeopathic medicine, especially if frequently repeated, are, as a rule, very destructive. Not infrequently, they endanger the patient's life or make his disease almost incurable ... (emphasis added).

Again the homeopath can clearly see in this aphorism how Hahnemann makes a distinction between dose and potency. In view of Hahnemann's words, I wonder how so many homeopaths can have their patients repeat daily doses of highly potentized remedies, advising the patient to, "Repeat the dose every day and come back when the bottle is empty." Read and reread **Aphorism 276** in its totality and may it be your guide in practice!

Susceptibility of the Patient

How to choose the right potency is the real question. The effect of the potency depends on the **susceptibility** of the particular patient, as outlined by Hahnemann:

A 281 ... for patients in whom one observes considerable sensitivity, the doses are increased far more slowly, and by far smaller amounts than for patients who are less sensitive, for whom the doses can be more rapidly increased. There are patients who are unusually sensitive, a thousand times more sensitive than those who are least sensitive.

In order to give correct guidelines for choosing the potency, I need to define what susceptibility means! **Susceptibility** is the capacity of the living organism to react to external and internal stimuli. In other words, it reflects the **reactivity** of the Vital Force (VF).

We feel pain on being pinched, we feel morose when something bad happens to us, excited when something good happens, etc. The idiosyncratic susceptibility of people is frequently seen when they are exposed to varying climates: one person will thrive in warm weather while others become sick. Altitude will affect some individuals very little and others adversely. Being at the seashore improves one person's condition while it makes another person sick. Mountainous regions are desired by some while avoided by others.

The power of assimilation and nutrition is another expression of susceptibility. Patients needing *Natrum carbonicum* and *Calcarea carbonica* do not assimilate milk (aggravation from milk), while patients needing *Arsenicum* and *Chelidonium* improve from it. And, of course, certain people are able to make wonderful contributions to a homeopathic drug proving when given a particular remedy whereas other provers will show no reaction whatsoever to the same substance. All these responses have to do with susceptibility.

The homeopath can derive from these examples, and especially from the definition of susceptibility, that one must avoid using any agent or anything in nature that would diminish, suppress, or destroy this power of susceptibility (reactivity) as this is the organism's natural defensive reaction. The status of a person's health (VF) determines their ability to react. If susceptibility is low, the VF has little reactivity, in other words, it can't react strongly in a secondary curative reaction (Aphorism 64). But if susceptibility is high, the VF can react in a strong, quick manner; this shows that the patient has a responsive defense system.

In disease, susceptibility or reactivity is exaggerated (if the person hasn't suppressed his "immune system" or if the VF is highly alerted), and the homeopath must be careful not to impair the body's ability to respond, because it is through this exaggerated reaction (a defensive reaction) that we find our clue to the simillimum. This exaggerated reaction or "throwing up" of symptoms is what the homeopath will use to find a remedy. Only the simillimum can satisfy the susceptibility, anything else will palliate or perhaps even suppress.

The VF reacts (and the question will be: to what extent?) against the entry of any "pathogenic factor" or disease-causing factor and tries to prevent mistunement through this reaction. There is no susceptibility in the dead; a dead person does not react to any stimulus. Partial destruction of the reactivity of the body by true organic lesions may render the patient a chronic invalid with impossibility of cure. With the destruction of susceptibility, the corresponding destruction of bacteria in infections is not accomplished, and the patient remains an invalid. In fact, that is why most severely diseased patients (those suffering from cancer, for instance) succumb to an infection and not to their chronic disease. Producing passive immunity through the use of sera (vaccinations) and even the use of antiseptics destroys normal susceptibility. One can see the same when antipyretics are used in feverish conditions. Their use retards the formation of antibodies, reduces the number of white blood cells (macrophages), and delays the body's ability to respond to an infection. The physician should remember Hippocrates' dictum: "Give me fever, and I cure any disease!" Fever is a manifestation of the vital reaction or susceptibility and thus of resistance to disease on the part of the organism. It is Nature's way of protecting the organism. The homeopath can formulate the potency choice when taking into account the patient's susceptibility as follows:

Susceptibility depends on the strength of the VF: low VF (lowered susceptibility) will necessitate a smaller stimulus or a lower potency since a higher potency would overwhelm the VF. When the VF is strong (strong susceptibility), the patient needs a higher stimulus or potency.

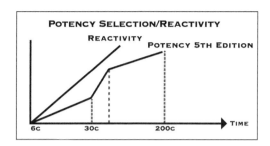

You can imagine that in the case of a long-term chronic illness or serious pathology, as well as in cases of great overload of miasmatic taint, the VF is not very susceptible or reactive. It is smothered. So should the homeopath stimulate it with a high potency? **No!** This VF is initially too sluggish to react!

I'd like to make this crystal clear to the reader. Take, for example, concentration camp survivors or shipwreck survivors who have been deprived of food and drink for a long time. What happens if they suddenly eat and drink too much, that is, the amount that would be normal for someone else? Many die, as the small intestine has shriveled and cannot absorb that amount of food or drink! (Note that it is not the stomach that has this function.) So to help these unfortunate victims, one needs to first feed them small quantities of food and drink in order to revive their susceptibility or reactivity—in other words, their capacity to absorb food again. Only then can they again consume normal quantities. How rapidly can they readapt? It depends on each individual—the length of time they were deprived of nourishment; their constitution, etc. Once their VF (or small intestines in this example) is restored, if one were to continue feeding them small quantities, they would barely be kept alive and could possibly die. These same principles must be applied in homeopathy!

Analogous to shipwreck survivors, if the VF, which was initially overwhelmed by the natural disease, has been slowly brought back to life through the judicious repetition of remedies in low potencies, then the reactivity or susceptibility of the VF will increase.

If the homeopath wants to follow Aphorism 2 and "expedite a permanent, **rapid** cure," when he sees that there is a positive reaction, the increased susceptibility of the patient will now warn him that he can and must jump to a higher potency. At this point, the VF **needs** a higher potency to react, especially if the homeopath does not see any further progress on lower potencies.

Let's say the homeopath sees a good reaction until the patient finishes a 6C RSB, and the patient feels much stronger. He should not hesitate to jump to 30C, using the 5th edition split-dose method. If the improved VF (just as in the survivors' case) were now stimulated with a 9C or 12C, it would be too small a stimulus to allow as rapid progress as can be achieved. The danger also exists that in the meantime another new or already existing, stronger pathogenic factor might overwhelm the VF because it is not well enough supported! Yes, the homeopath could still see progress, but not as fast as he otherwise might. There are exceptions. The homeopath sometimes finds in the practice, when a patient does well on the C scale, that after 30C, switching to LMs gives less progress, not always more. In those cases it is better to stimulate the VF using a 200C split dose! For some unknown reason, some patients do better on C potencies than on LM potencies! On the other hand, I have had striking results after one single dose of LM potency, where the C scale did nothing.

MIASMATIC BLOCK

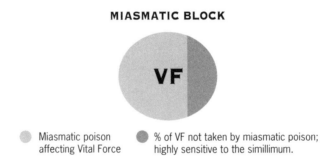

● Miasmatic poison affecting Vital Force

● % of VF not taken by miasmatic poison; highly sensitive to the simillimum.

Fine-Tuning This Method

Often in the practice, for example, the patient is initially doing very well on a 6C split dose for their chronic disease. Then halfway through the RSB, the patient suddenly stops going forward or there is barely any change or progress perceptible. Rather than **first** thinking of a miasmatic block, consider that the susceptibility of your patient's VF has perhaps increased and needs a stronger stimulus (higher potency) to make the cure go forward. On going to 30C the homeopath sees the case going forward again. This in fact corresponds to what Kent always said, when his colleagues asked his advice regarding stuck cases: "Increase the potency!" What the homeopath aims toward is that the potency selection follows the increase in reactivity, so both lines must run parallel in order to achieve a cure.

—

A hereditary component and a general adaptability combine in determining susceptibility. Susceptibility can be modified under various circumstances, even by intrauterine events as well as by environment, sickness, mode of living, occupation, diet, etc. (Aphorism 77). Traditional Chinese Medicine (TCM) acknowledges the various emotions, foods, climate, tastes, etc. that influence each organ. As discussed in Chapter 13 on intrauterine questions, even the age of the parents at the moment of conception will determine the quality of the VF and thus the susceptibility of the newborn. In other words, susceptibility is not fixed but influenced by many factors. No definite criteria exist for measuring susceptibility yet the occurrence of the disease and its cure depend on recognizing varying levels of susceptibility, as they will influence the choice of potency.

When exposed to excessive cold, wind, dampness, or any perverse Qi recognized by TCM (or the telluric and meteorological factors discussed in Aphorism 73), anyone can get sick. But if someone becomes sick when exposed to the slightest draft, then the homeopath should presume that this person has a heightened susceptibility to this climate factor. **A person becomes easily vulnerable to diseases that are linked to causative factors to which he is particularly susceptible**, for example, cold, wind, dampness, etc. So according to TCM, someone gets frequent colds and flu because he is susceptible to invasion of Wind-Cold. Or a patient with rheumatic problems experiences flare-ups when exposed to Cold-Dampness (except *Causticum*). Similarly, when a remedy is administered to healthy persons (i.e., in provings), those who are susceptible to that particular drug will be most affected and will exhibit more symptoms (i.e., proving symptoms).

As to the process of cure, the homeopath depends much upon the susceptibility of the patient's VF. In the absence of requisite or adequate susceptibility (e.g., low VF in a dying patient), we cannot possibly effect cure with highly potentized remedies. In homeopathy, susceptibility most clearly influences the selection of potency. The general rule is:

The greater the patient's susceptibility, the higher the selected potency.

As usual there will be exceptions, for example:

The closer the chosen remedy is to the simillimum and the more susceptible the diseased organ, the higher the advisable potency.

—

Dr. von Boenninghausen expressed it in almost the same way:

> The more receptive the organism, the higher the potency and the smaller the dose must be (von Boenninghausen, 1991, p. 146).

Note that von Boenninghausen clearly distinguishes between dose and potency!

Ascertaining the Degree of Susceptibility in a Patient

No definite criteria exist, and I don't believe it is possible to put forward a general rule for determining the patient's susceptibility. As usual, one should not use "cookbook" or protocol-type prescribing! That said, certain observations and factors can help us as we will see in the following examples.

Most failures in the practice occur not because of a wrong remedy selection but because of wrong potency and dose selection, in addition to not being able to understand the correct management in follow-up visits. In general, the homeopath can stick to "30C split dose for chronic diseases" for starters. The bigger question is: at what point does the homeopath move to LMs or to higher C-scale potencies? Or, in what cases can the homeopath start with an even higher C-scale potency?

In *acute* diseases, the homeopath should still use 200C and 1M potencies via the split-dose method. It is the potency choice in chronic diseases that needs fine-tuning. I shall attempt to set down some logical guidelines for potency selection in most clinical cases.

• First, there are three classes of patients that **always require low potencies: hypersensitive patients**, patients with **extensive physical pathology**, and patients with **suppressed skin diseases**. Although the hypersensitive patient's susceptibility is the highest, a very high potency will prove harmful. The reactivity of a hypersensitive patient is always on high alert. Such a person behaves like a nervous race horse that needs only a small stimulus to explode from the starting gate. For all these patients, the homeopath should always start with a 6C potency of his chosen simillimum and administer a minimum amount of remedy for the test dose. To do this, dissolve 1 pellet of the remedy in an 8-oz. RSB (see *Achieving and Maintaining the Simillimum*, p.35, for instructions on preparing an RSB). Then instruct the patient to take the test dose as follows:

1. **Do not** succuss the RSB for the first dose (your test dose).

2. Dilute 2 to 3 drops of the remedy from the RSB in 4 oz. of purified water.

3. Vigorously stir the solution.

—

4. Take 2 to 3 drops from the 4-oz. cup. This is your test dose.

5. Call me 3 days after the test dose to evaluate your response.

For subsequent doses, add only 2 succussions with each successive dose. As the VF gets stronger, you can add more succussions, for example, 0 succussions added to the test dose, 2 succussions added to the second dose, 4 succussions added to the third dose, and so on. This can be done as the patient is steadily improving and as long as they experience no aggravation. When dealing with these patients, this gentle method **supersedes any other consideration** because you will avoid severe similar aggravations, which can lead to patients' abandoning homeopathic care. Remember, **always use a low potency and low dose when starting to treat skin diseases that were suppressed for a long time** with cortisone. Higher doses and potencies will cause not only a similar aggravation but also an accelerated exteriorization of the internal imbalance. While the homeopathic remedy stimulates this exteriorization, it must proceed in a manner tolerable for the patient. No patient will consider exteriorization beneficial when he suffers from more severe itching or burning, from loss of sleep, and from a spreading of his lesions to the point of disfigurement.

What other classes of patients we can assign a potency choice to?

• For a person whose nerves seem to be strong (i.e., not a neurotic, hysterical person with frail nerves but rather a person who is emotionally well-adjusted), a dose of 1M or 10M may be required. That does not mean that in these cases a 6C or 30C would not do anything; it will stimulate the VF but not to the point that the patient might be able note it! A cure may be achieved by using a lower potency than required but only if the dose is repeated again and again. This brings a danger to the practice. In these cases, it might initially look like there is no improvement and this may often lead to faulty decisions on the part of the homeopath: to change the remedy, to use nosodes for presumed miasmatic blocks, etc. Certainly it will have delayed the cure and will not meet the Aphorism 2 stipulation of "a **rapid cure**"!

In provings and when under-dosing, a single dose of a potentized remedy may not be able to produce any change (unless the person is hypersensitive), but if that low-potency remedy is repeated several times, symptoms will definitely be produced (when conducting a proving) or symptoms will start improving (in clinical cases). **If the same stimulus is repeated, the susceptibility or reactivity will increase!** It is like reviving a very weak person. For that reason, as the patient's reactivity increases, the VF requires a stronger potency to move the case forward and to further cure the patient, even when the natural disease has decreased after repetition of judiciously chosen remedy doses. The "stronger person" or the state of "increased susceptibility" asks for, even demands, a stronger stimulus because a stimulus that is too gentle can hardly be felt by the patient.

• The homeopath must differentiate between "**dynamic pathology**" and "**organic pathology**." The time from the start of the disease up to the onset of organic changes is considered "dynamic" pathology. On the other hand, the descriptions in pathology text books or in a *Merck Manual* are of organic pathology. In the earlier stage of dynamic pathology, the patient's susceptibility is still high (his VF is still strong), and he will respond to a high potency, though you still have to use the 5th edition or LMs (6th edition) and a test dose to determine the right interval of repetition. For example, in a case of sycotic hypertension with no organic lesions and where lab tests (Cr, BUN, lipid profile, fibrinogen, etc.) are within normal range, even if this condition has been present for 10 years and more, use a higher potency! **Always give a test dose!** Even when switching from a lower potency to a higher one, the homeopath must first do a test dose. Don't just continue with the same dose size and/or frequency of repetition that you had used before! The susceptibility may already have increased, and in that case, you can increase the potency and dose (e.g., increase the number of succussions, increase the dose from drops to teaspoons, etc).

• Highly susceptible patients are also those affected by the increasing number of **neurotic ailments or persons suffering from various so-called mental disorders**. These patients are very susceptible to acute diseases (contrary some psychiatrists' assertion that schizophrenics do not get acute diseases), so these cases will only be resolved by minute doses of a high potency. If the homeopath uses a 6C potency, the repetition of such low potency will lead to an increase of the natural disease, for example, neurotic or mental expressions. Imagine a patient with suicidal ideation: the homeopath bombards him with repeated doses of 6C potency! What will happen? Another danger is that too frequent repetition of too low a potency will create many accessory symptoms, which will push these patients to the brink of incurability.

• Low potencies should be used where the susceptibility is low: for instance in established paralysis (hemiplegia, post-status stroke, brain or spinal tumor, paraplegia). These are caused by destruction of nerves (as are cases of multiple sclerosis), thus true organic pathology is present and the rule of using low potencies remains valid. Other such diseases are numerous: Parkinson's disease, amyotrophic lateral sclerosis, severe rheumatoid arthritis, insulin-dependent diabetes, etc.

• On the other hand, if paralysis is caused by inflammation (**psoric phase**) and no organic changes exist, the susceptibility remains high, so a high potency can be used. In cases of Bell's palsy and epilepsy, repetition of high potencies, even in older cases, yields unexpectedly good results. In these cases, LM potencies will be the best!

• In chronic cases of cholera, severe diarrhea, and prolonged profuse bleeding: the VF and susceptibility are low, requiring low potencies!

• In case of tumors, warts, and other growths, lower potencies in the beginning and, as soon as result is noticed, administer higher potencies. In case of tumors, the susceptibility remains high. (A tumor is the end result of dynamic pathology.)

• Susceptibility of children is usually greater than that of adults, hence if there is no gross organic pathology, high or medium potencies yield better results (LMs, 200C, and higher).

• The susceptibility of a patient with a **long-term chronic disease** gradually diminishes as a result of long suffering, so it is better in such cases to start with low potencies (6C).

• Susceptibility decreases if there are pathological changes in both acute and chronic cases, so start with low potencies!

• Susceptibility decreases in diseases affecting vital organs—kidneys, eyes, heart, pancreas, lungs, brain, etc.—so use low potencies!

• Then there is the **problem of idiosyncrasy**, a special form of increased susceptibility! This is a peculiar corporeal constitution which is dangerously affected by exposure to an apparently inert or otherwise harmless substance (peanuts, strawberries, crustaceans, etc.) For example, everyone likes the smell of a rose. Yet, I have had patients who would literally taste the rose in their mouth and even faint from it. This occurs when someone has a peculiar hyper-susceptibility to roses. So idiosyncrasy is a constitutional defect and affects both the mental and physical spheres simultaneously. These cases are very difficult to cure except by using the **olfaction** method via split dosing in low potencies. Remember that although these patients possess high susceptibility, they are hypersensitive. Such patients are of course very useful for remedy provings. If the homeopath wants to find out the full drug picture of a remedy, he should choose this kind of person for a proving!

Note that, **in my experience, it is absolutely contrary to our guidelines** *to prescribe low potencies (6C) for acute illnesses!*

—

POTENCY SELECTION — APHORISM 281

HIGHER POTENCY SELECTION	LOWER POTENCY SELECTION
1. NATURE OF DISEASE	
HIGH SUSCEPTIBILITY/REACTIVITY	**LOW REACTIVITY**
Sudden onset, rapid pace	Gradual onset, slow pace
Functional, reversible/dynamic	Structural, irreversible
2. ETIOLOGY	
Acute/sudden	Chronic
3. MIASM	
(Nosodes do not correlate with potency selections)	
Psora, Tubercular	Sycosis, Syphilitic
4. SYMPTOMS	
Many characteristic symptoms	Few symptoms: One-sided disease
Predominance of individual symptoms	Predominance of pathognomic symptoms
5. DEGREE OF SIMILARITY	
The closer to the simillimum—	Distant Simile
the SMALLER the DOSE and the	
HIGHER the POTENCY	
6. SUPPRESSION	
—	Always LOWER
7. NATURE OF PERSON	
Children, vigorous, non-addicted person,	Old age, sluggish
predominantly M/E	addicted, one-sided
8. VITALITY	
Strong	Low

A Great Question Regarding Dose

One of my best students asked me a great question regarding dose and potency after reading my book, *Achieving and Maintaining the Simillimum*.

Student's dilemma: "I've been wrestling with a problem concerning homeopathic philosophy and so far the problem is winning. We know that our remedies become more powerful and deeper acting the more they are diluted and the more they are succussed (De Schepper, 2004, pp. 30-31). Hahnemann states in the 5th edition of the *Organon* (R.E. Dudgeon's translation) that:

> **A 286** The effect of a homeopathic dose of medicine increases, the greater the quantity of fluid in which it is dissolved when administered to the patient.

"Since greater dilution increases the power of a remedy, isn't a pellet diluted in 8 oz. of water MORE powerful than a pellet diluted in 4 oz. of water (assuming each dilution receives an equal number of succussions)? Yet, for normally

—

sensitive patients we dissolve a pellet of the remedy in a 4-oz. RSB and for hypersensitive patients we dissolve a pellet of the remedy in an 8-oz. RSB.

"I'm confused by what Hahnemann says in the 5th edition of the *Organon*:

> **A 286** Although theorists may imagine that there should be a weakening of the action of the dose of medicine by its dilution with a large quantity of liquid, experience asserts exactly the opposite …

"What am I missing or forgetting here? I'm sure that somewhere in the *Organon* there's a clear and easy resolution to my conundrum, and I'm equally sure that my brain is too tied up in knots at the moment to be able to see it."

Dr. Luc' answer: "When I discussed Aphorism 286 of the **5th** edition of the *Organon* in *Achieving and Maintaining the Simillimum*, it was to demonstrate that Hahnemann used diluted doses. I am afraid that, by not giving more explanation, this can indeed sound contradictory! The whole story starts at Aphorism 275 and continues until Aphorism 293 of the **5th edition of the *Organon*.** In these aphorisms Hahnemann speaks about the minimum **dose**.

"When you read Aphorism 286 by itself it seems to create some confusion. However, when the homeopath looks at the whole story, he must differentiate between the amount of water in the **RSB** and **the size of the dose** (e.g., drops, teaspoons, etc.) **given to the patient**. Indeed, the homeopath will dilute the remedy more if he puts it into an 8-oz. RSB instead of a 4-oz. RSB, but Aphorism 286 is not referring to the amount of water used to dilute a pellet in the RSB. Aphorism 286 is referring to the **dose administered to the patient**.

"The dose given to the patient is a different matter. Let's assume the homeopath gives **one drop as a dose** to the patient (either from the RSB or, in even more diluted form, from the first cup). Hahnemann always talks about the **minuteness of the dose** because it comes into contact with a great surface of sensitive nerves (Aphorism 286, 5th edition):

> **A 286** For in this case, when the medicine is taken, it comes in contact with a much larger surface of sensitive nerves responsive to the medicinal action (Dudgeon, 2001, p. 147).

"Besides the smallest possible dose, there is a second component that Hahnemann teaches us in these aphorisms. In Aphorism 281, in a footnote to the 5th edition, Hahnemann states that:

> **A 281** The inherent power of medicinal substances is so powerful in character that of late years I have been compelled by experience to reduce the **ten** successions to **two** (Ibid, 2001, p. 143).

"The bottom line is that a larger amount of liquid in the RSB will dilute the strength of the remedy. When the homeopath is dealing with **sensitive** patients, the patient should not succuss the 8-oz. RSB for the test dose. Then the patient should dilute **2 to 3 drops** of remedy from the RSB in a 4-oz. cup of purified water, and then the patient should take **2 to 3 drops** from that the 4-oz. cup. This **results in fewer nerve endings being touched**, in comparison with a teaspoon-sized dose, for instance. Giving a teaspoon or tablespoon from the cup as a dose on the patient's tongue will affect more nerve endings and that dose will have a stronger effect. This is not a problem when treating *acute* diseases. The VF can handle and requests such a potent dose in those cases."

I want to mention here that, when going from the 5th to the 6th edition of the *Organon*, Hahnemann replaced many aphorisms. Indeed Aphorism 286 of the 6th edition of the *Organon* says nothing about this but mentions only magnetism and family. Aphorisms 280, 281, 282, and 283 are entirely rewritten in the 6th edition. Aphorisms 284 and 286 are entirely omitted in 6th edition.

By extensively studying **the differences** between the 5th and the 6th editions of the *Organon*, I also came upon some astute observations of Hahnemann's that should be brought to the homeopath's attention. "Eminent" homeopaths who treat cancer claim that several doses of several different remedies are advisable in the first weeks of cancer treatment because such a condition is considered an "emergency" or an "acute" situation. Let's look at that claim in detail and in relation to what Hahnemann wrote.

First of all, cancer is a *chronic*, mixed miasmatic state and should be approached like any other chronic case. Secondly, the VF of such patients is inherently mistuned and decreased in strength, so that they have become "sensitive" patients with very serious pathology. All the more reason to approach these cases with great care and with a single remedy in small dose and low potency! This is what Hahnemann had to say in a footnote to the 5th edition of the *Organon*:

A 293 *Imperfect* homeopaths who think themselves monstrously clever, not infrequently deluge their patients in difficult cases with doses of different medicines, given rapidly one after the other, which although they *might have been homeopathically selected* (emphasis added), and given in highly potentized attenuation, bring the patient in such overexcited state that life and death are struggling for the mastery and the least additionally quantity of medicine would infallible kill them (Ibid, 2001, p. 153).

What a condemnation of such prescribing techniques! Forget "cookbook prescribing," which goes against all the principles of Hahnemannian homeopathy!

—

How I Select the Potency and Dose in My Practice

Over the last few years I have fine-tuned my approach to giving a remedy. Some people think this has do with a lack of results or a wavering and waffling of my opinion regarding potency and dose selection. On the contrary, I have been consumed with a desire to follow Hahnemann's advice in Aphorism 2—to restore health in the most gentle, permanent, and rapid manner. On-going research in my homeopathic practice continually forces me to fully understand what Hahnemann says. And in my attempt to follow Hahnemann's words, my patients are daily reminders of how I can improve the results we get on their healing path. The *Organon* is my trusted source and has never disappointed me.

Here is my present approach for treating **chronic** diseases. These techniques, based on Hahnemann's 5th and 6th editions of the *Organon*, have worked well for everything that I have discussed in this chapter.

I always start with a 30C potency unless the patient is a true hypersensitive, has extensive physical pathology, or has a suppressed skin disease (see the section above: "Ascertaining the Degree of Susceptibility in a Patient"). For these special cases I start with a 6C. Even if I start with a 30C in cases of true hypersensitivity or true pathology, I can adjust the dose immediately if it's too strong for the patient.

I put 1 pellet of the patient's remedy in an 8-oz. RSB (see *Achieving and Maintaining the Simillimum* for instructions, p. 35). I instruct the patient to take a test dose as follows:

1. **Do not** succuss the RSB for the first dose (your test dose).

2. Dilute __ teaspoon of the remedy from the RSB in 4 oz. of purified water.

3. Vigorously stir the solution.

4. Take __ teaspoon from the 4-oz. cup. This is your test dose.

5. Call me 3 days after the test dose to evaluate your response.

Why a 30C potency? No matter what chronic problem I am treating, in almost all cases it is easy to adjust the potency (thanks to the succussions). If the patient's response was too intense, I immediately reduce the dose and only add 1 succussion for the next dose. If the patient's response was insufficient, then I can increase the succussions from 2 to 10.

I always ask the patient to report back to me the third day after this test dose to judge their reaction. The patient waits three days and does not repeat the

—

remedy until we have evaluated their response. If a good reaction is seen, as is frequently the case with this potency and dose of the well-selected homeopathic remedy, I will immediately increase the potency by adding 2 succussions and **reduce the dose to drops**! For the second dose, I instruct the patient to:

1. Succuss the RSB 2 times.

2. Dilute 2 to 3 drops of the remedy from the RSB in 4 oz. of purified water.

3. Vigorously stir the solution.

4. Take 2 to 3 drops from the 4-oz. cup.

Following the dictum that I have set forth in this chapter, I will almost never have to increase the dose but can speed up the process by increasing the potency, first by adding succussions to the 30C RSB. And then, often, by increasing the potency from a 30C to a 200C or LM1 even before the patient finishes the 30C RSB. I have seen so many patients blossom when treated in this fashion, and they are very grateful that no awful aggravations occur during this process.

Here's a tip about repeating the remedy or determining the interval between doses. The initial interval is determined after the test dose. If no spectacular improvement is seen (Aphorism 246), then initially—that is, for the next 14 days—I let the patient repeat the remedy every other day. However, this advice needs to be given with caution. First, when I evaluate the response with the patient on the third day after the test dose, I tell them that if any of their symptoms aggravate during the next 10 days, they are to call me immediately. Then I always check back in with the patient on day 10. I explain to the patient that the intervals between doses will change throughout the process of cure. For example, as the potency increases, the healthier and more reactive VF can often "run" longer with each dose. **The interval between doses can change continuously as the patient progresses.**

I also explain to the patient that if something related to the remedy happens in their life, the remedy can be used up faster and therefore the interval between doses will be shortened. Take the case of *Sepia*, for instance. The patient can do very well on well-chosen doses but suddenly more demands (work, holidays, etc.) are put on the *Sepia* patient. The remedy will be used up more quickly. Therefore, I find it imperative from the beginning (at time of the first consult) to determine with the patient the parameters or **indicators** belonging to his case. These indicators will help patients ascertain their progress and determine when they need to repeat their remedy.

Let's look at the *Sepia* example again. The patient presents with fatigue in the afternoon necessitating a nap. She is irritable and curt when fatigued and has dizzy spells that occur with lower back pains. All these and other expressions can act as guidelines. They show us how well the remedy is working, and even more importantly, they let us know when to repeat the dose. This is different from the 4th edition dry dose method because when using the 5th or 6th edition *Organon* methods, we can repeat the remedy more often (see guidelines in Aphorism 246). In my experience, the patient understands this explanation very well and feels in control of his destiny and involved in his cure, which is psychologically important!

Every day in my practice I see how important a role the size of the dose (the minimum dose!) plays. Two drops may be perfect, one drop may be too little, three drops may create a similar aggravation! Let no homeopath doubt this! I see botched cases every day in my practice. When the remedy is correctly selected by the homeopath (the right name, e.g., *Sepia*), but the potency and dose are not carefully considered, then a great similar aggravation occurs (which is often welcomed by the homeopath, but not by the patient). In addition, I often see the homeopath repeating the same potency many more times, which then leads to the development of accessory symptoms and eventually, incurability! Please do not follow the advice of the "master teacher" who says, "only the name of the remedy" not the potency or dose is important!

Chapter 15: Miasms Revisited

Modern Findings and Problems

The 2006 death from complications of anorexia of a 21-year-old Brazilian model, Ana Carolina Reston, not only reignited the debate about the fashion industry and eating disorders, but brought to light again the many questions that allopathy still has about etiology, in particular, the role of genes in such disorders and others. Allopathy indicts genes, early environmental influences, family variables, and often a "precipitating event"—the homeopathic Never Well Since (NWS) event—as culpable factors in such cases. According to allopathy, in cases of anorexia, genes create a gun; the fashion industry, the modern image of "perfection", and environmental factors, load the gun. The "trigger" is pulled by an "emotional distress." Homeopaths have dealt with this terminology since 1816. For the homeopath, genes are understood via miasms and triggers may be emotional, physical (e.g., head trauma), or mental (e.g., mental overwork). Where we homeopaths differ from allopaths is that we are not stalled in terms of understanding. Over the last 200 years, homeopathy has offered the means (remedies) to provide an individual approach, which is just about the only way a cure can be obtained in such cases.

Psychiatrists claim, "One does not become anorexic because one wants to." They claim that a growing body of research supports genetic and biological pieces to the puzzle. A 2005 study conducted by the University of Pittsburgh School of Medicine identified six core traits that appear to be linked to genes associated with both anorexia and bulimia: obsessive behavior, age of first menstruation, anxiety, lifetime minimum body-mass index, concern over mistakes, and food-related obsessions.

To me this sounds like the typical allopathic approach: put common traits into a category, label it as an "acceptable" disease, then use the disease label to diagnose those unfortunate souls with a few symptoms linked to that disease. But does allopathy possess medications that address the many different mental/emotional factors and make the patient move forward as his "terrain" is changed? Not at all! Their psychotropic medications usually rob the patient of the small remnant of psychological freedom he possesses, condemning him to a robotic life of indifference, void of feelings. This surely cannot be called a cure.

—

Interesting, too, was a study of twins with anorexia, carried out at the University of North Carolina and the Karolinska Institute in Stockholm, which concluded that genetic makeup could account for more than half the risk of developing an eating disorder. The homeopath looks at this in an entirely different way. Twins *and* anorexia nervosa are different expressions of the same root, the syphilitic miasm. While the correlation found in this study is astronomical, the figure would be much higher if, in the family history of these twins, other expressions of the syphilitic miasm were taken into account: alcoholism, mental disease, suicide, destructive illnesses like advanced diabetes or insulin-dependent diabetes, multiple sclerosis, Alzheimer's, ALS (Lou Gehrig's disease), and a whole slew of autoimmune disorders. While million-dollar studies are currently looking for specific genes that lead to susceptibility to anorexia or to other of the above-mentioned diseases, my question to allopathy is this: "When you find that gene, what are you going to do about it? Replace it? Why was it defective in the first place?" Allopathy has mapped many genes linked to diseases but so far the therapeutic result of that work is zero!

Here is another statistic for anorexia: people with anorexia are 56 times more likely than their peers to commit suicide. This only confirms the homeopathic theory of miasms: anorexia is an expression of the syphilitic miasm and occurs in people with the presence of this miasmatic taint in the family history. Allopathy has still a long way to go before it recognizes such a relationship.

Other heroic allopathic interventions bring the need of intrauterine or better, pre-conception genetic therapy. Eugenics changes the DNA pattern before pregnancy to assure a healthy outcome of the pregnancy. Recently, attention to the need for such intervention was accentuated by the plight of a bedridden 9-year-old girl named Ashley. She was born with static encephalopathy or severe brain damage. In fact, it was predicted that she would never go beyond the intellect of an 18-month-old infant. In a case fraught with ethical questions, the parents have stunted her growth to keep their little "pillow angel," as they call her, a manageable and more portable size. This young girl had her uterus and breast tissue removed and received large doses of hormones to halt her growth. These parents have chosen an extremely slippery slope, although I do not doubt their good intentions. Such a choice can set a precedent: "Should we deal with children with permanent behavioral problems by putting them into permanent childhood?" I am not denying the struggle thousands of parents face to care for severely disabled children as they grow up. Interventions such as the one in Ashley's case border on mutilation and appear inhumane. Why then does allopathy refuse to study homeopathy more closely? In my opinion, cases such as these indicate a syphilitic miasmatic expression that will likely be found in the

—

parents. This syphilitic expression could have been avoided if both parents had received excellent homeopathic treatment before conceiving their daughter. I fear that it will remain a pipe dream that allopathy will open its doors to implementing homeopathy, even though doing so would mean that many challenged children could be born without serious problems. Homeopathic intervention before conception and even during the pregnancy could spare a lot of needless trauma.

Homeopathic intervention is even more crucial in the autism spectrum disorder (ASD) epidemic. In the near future and even now, many people will be forced to accept a struggle with life as autistic adults or as parents of autistic adults. This future tidal wave of a maturing autistic population will soon overwhelm not only the emotional and financial resources of families, but Medicaid and government social services budgets.

What is really at the heart of this debate? What has caused autism rates to increase so much in less than 20 years? Better diagnosis? Preposterous! The epidemic is *real* and cannot be explained by saying that the diagnostic skills of doctors suddenly improved in the late 1990s. A more logical suggestion is that something changed in the 1990s. The number of mercury-containing vaccines given to children tripled in the 1990s, to give just one factor. Homeopaths already know the root cause. In Chapter 3, I explained how the common symptoms of ASD all point to the syphilitic miasm. The homeopath can therefore expect that mercury-laden vaccines would be a serious trigger for all those children with a syphilitic family background, thus increasing the risk for ASD. Mercury or *Mercurius* is one of the greatest anti-syphilitic remedies!

I read a remark from a well-meaning allopathic physician who said, "This epidemic cannot be due to the sudden activation of a mystery gene in hundreds of thousands of children." She does not realize that she is actually denying the truth of the matter. Homeopaths know that a dormant (latent) miasmatic state can be aroused by many triggers. These triggers **do** in fact activate the dormant gene! And vaccinations are not the only triggers. Emotions, lifestyle, diet, physical stressors, and mental triggers can activate latent miasmatic states at any time!

Origin of Miasmatic Theory

One hundred years after Hahnemann, the Frenchman Trousseau introduced the term *diathesis*, which is remarkably similar to the idea formulated by Hahnemann. Trousseau said, "It is the individual's hereditary disposition to contract a particular group of illnesses."

In spite of earlier successes in practice, Hahnemann had found by 1816 that the treatment of true chronic illness with homeopathic remedies was first satisfactory, then less favorable, and always ended in hopelessness ... in other words no true cure of a chronic disease had been achieved at this point. Hahnemann says in *Chronic Diseases:*

> **CD** ... repeated fright, grief, sorrow and continuous vexation, often caused in a weakened body the re-appearance of one or more of the ailments which seemed to have been already overcome; and this condition was often aggravated by some quite new concomitants, which if not more threatening than the former ones which had been removed homeopathically were often just as troublesome and now more obstinate. ... the remedy which had been serviceable the first time would prove less useful, and when repeated again it would help still less ... new symptoms of the disease would be added which could be removed only inadequately and imperfectly ... (1997, Vol. 1, p. 3).

Only by putting into practice the miasmatic theory he first wrote about in the year 1827 was Hahnemann able to cure chronic diseases. This should be a warning to all homeopaths: as explained in *Hahnemann Revisited* (De Schepper, 1999, p. 197), a perfect prescription is not just the totality of the symptoms according to Aphorism 7—the simillimum in the eyes of many homeopaths. We *must* add Aphorism 5 in which Hahnemann talks about constitution, lifestyle, hygiene, and *predisposition* or miasms. If the homeopath considers all the patient's symptoms but not the miasmatic background, he can never claim that the entire totality has been considered. It is not only useful but in fact indispensable to diagnose the dominant miasmatic state in each and every one of our patients.

Defining the patient by his miasms gives us distinct advantages. First, if the miasm is not considered, what the homeopath chooses as the simillimum will turn out to be merely palliative or at best a remedy that works superficially to remove some symptoms but never truly prevents recurrence of the natural illness or the resurgence of a new disease. Secondly, knowing the predominant miasmatic state of the patient enables the homeopath to understand the profound pathology that he inevitably must confront sooner or later and which it is his duty to bring to the surface, so that it will be accessible to the correct treatment. Thirdly, this knowledge gives us an unshakeable basis for the *prognosis* of the case. Obviously, the structure-deforming sycotic and syphilitic miasmatic states are worse than the physiological changes that occur in the psoric miasm. Very importantly, a chronic miasmatic disease left uncured will automatically be transmitted to the next generation. At this point, the homeopath alone is able to stop this vicious cycle. The progression of the patient's case from one miasmatic state to another also tells the homeopath whether he is following Hering's Set of Observations (see Chap. 16). If, after the remedy, the patient's symptoms go from syphilitic ones to sycotic ones, then this is a proof of the right remedy. It can mean that the first predominantly syphilitic layer has been resolved and the sycotic layer, which was suspended, has now become active. Either way, it is a sign of good progress. Therefore, taking Aphorisms 5 and 7 into account in solving a case is a *must*.

Let's take a simple example. Let's say the homeopath has a patient with the following symptoms: irritability, slowness in answering questions, abundant salivation, ineffectual stools, ciliary blepharitis, pain in the throat as if an apple core was sticking in it, pressing and stitching pain in the liver that is worse at night, crooked teeth, aversion to meat, and a sweetish taste in the mouth. The practitioner might recognize the remedy *Mercurius*. To the joy of the patient, *Mercurius* will alleviate some symptoms, but is it the simillimum?

Hahnemann's method demands more from the homeopath. If he investigates the patient more exhaustively, he will find further details that will change his mind about the prescription of *Mercurius*. The homeopath finds that the patient's mind is full of concerns about imaginary things that might happen to him; he feels anxiety about the present and the future; he is reserved although he desires company and wants to go home. It will be found that he fears he will lose his reason; or that people will observe his confusion of mind; or that he has anxiety about his spiritual welfare, and often talks to God. He is easily offended but rarely expresses it except through obstinate behavior. He is very much concerned about and tied to his family but easily exhausted by physical demands and those from mental work (thinking is difficult). His symptoms improve when he is kept occupied. Often he feels weariness in lower limbs and weeps when admonished. These are mostly psoric symptoms, so this is a patient with *predominant psora* and a touch of *syphilis*. Now we see that *Calcarea carbonica* is a much better choice for this patient, and, in fact, the simillimum for this patient was *Calcarea carbonica*. Giving *Calcarea carbonica* to this patient insures that Aphorisms 5 and 7 are addressed. *Calcarea carbonica* will be the most appropriate stimulus for the Vital Force (VF)—guiding the patient towards true homeostasis. I could classify this case miasmatically as being predominantly psoric and secondarily as luetic or syphilitic, indicated as "P/l" (i.e., capital "P" indicates the predominant psoric miasm and lowercase "l" indicates the secondary luetic or syphilitic miasm). This reflects the kind of miasmatic remedy needed to cure the case. The homeopath needs to research the proving symptoms and find a remedy that is "P/l" or mostly psoric and a little luetic! (See pp. 201-207 and the section: Denoting Miasmatic Tendencies of Clinical Expressions.)

The homeopath must also remember what Hahnemann writes in *Chronic Diseases*:

> **CD** But that the original malady sought for must be also of a *miasmatic*, chronic nature clearly appeared to me from this circumstance, that after it has once advanced and developed to a certain degree it can never be removed by the strength of any robust condition, it can never be overcome by the most wholesome diet and order of life, nor will it die out of itself. But it is evermore aggravated, from year to year, through a transition into other and more serious symptoms, even till the end of man's life, like every other chronic, miasmatic sickness ... (1997, Vol. 1, p. 6).

The miasm will remain smoldering in the organism, waiting for a decrease in strength of the VF, for moments of turmoil (e.g., puberty, menopause, etc.) to flare up and hinder the VF in its action geared toward defending the human organism against exterior and interior stimuli. Let me give the reader a small example from my practice to demonstrate the awakening of the latent miasm. I have seen this situation numerous times.

"This young man used to be of a quiet, good and timid disposition. Everything started around puberty. Now he desires to be left alone. He flies into a rage when he is told to do something and throws things around, hitting everything available. His father is in prison."

The homeopath can see the awakening of the syphilitic miasm, in this case at the time of puberty. All too often the public accepts this change in behavior as "raging hormones." What they don't know is that their child is exhibiting his miasmatic inheritance.

Miasmatic illness will only increase in strength over time, creating an ever more complex disease, leading the person slowly to the grave. The allopathic approach is to destroy the local expression, and this approach is very destructive. Hahnemann writes:

> **A 204** Apart from all the chronic troubles, complaints, and diseases arising from a prolonged unhealthy way of living (par. 77) and the innumerable chronic medicinal diseases (par. 74) arising from the unwise, persistent, violent, and pernicious treatment that the old school employs, often even for minor complaints, most chronic diseases develop from these three chronic miasms: internal syphilis, internal sycosis, but most of all, and to a disproportionate extent, internal psora.
>
> Each of these miasms has already occupied the entire organism and permeated all its parts before the appearance of the primary, vicarious local symptom (the scabies eruption in psora, the chancre or inguinal bubo in syphilis, and the fig-warts in sycosis), which prevents its full manifestation.

—

If these miasms are by external means deprived of the vicarious local symptoms that allay the general internal malady, sooner or later the characteristic disease that the Creator of nature has decreed for each of them must inevitably develop and manifest fully and thus spread all the nameless misery, the incredible multitude of chronic diseases, which have plagued the human race for hundreds and thousands of years.

None of them would have manifested themselves so often if physicians had wisely endeavored to cure these three miasms fundamentally and to extinguish them in the organism exclusively by the internal use of homeopathic medicines appropriate to each, *without disturbing their external symptoms through topical treatment* ... (emphasis added).

When will this ring a bell for today's allopaths when treating cancer? Nothing but *local* treatment is used, and it is up to the obstructed VF whether the patient will live or die, not to chemotherapy or radiation. As any other miasm, cancer makes the *whole* organism sick *immediately* and in a secondary attempt from the VF to ask for help, the body throws local symptoms to the surface to be seen (Aphorisms 201 to 202).

Hahnemann does call miasms "diathesis" in further aphorisms. As the homeopath understands now, a true diathesis is defined by a multitude of manifestations with the same origin. For more information, see *Hahnemann Revisited* (De Schepper, 1999, Part Three).

A Closer Study of the Basic Miasms

Nowadays, homeopaths seem to invent more and more miasms, as if homeopathy was not difficult enough to comprehend and practice. In *Hahnemann Revisited*, I discussed five different miasms—tubercular and cancer in addition to the three main miasms. I would now like to see if this miasmatic theory can be simplified and translated into a form that is easier to apply in practice. Since the choice of a deep-working remedy will depend on the homeopath's miasmatic knowledge, a fine-tuned definition and practical theory might be appropriate. The whole miasmatic issue has become more clear to me the more I taught and was confronted with clinical cases. I would like to have another go at explaining it.

It is always good to define exactly what we are dealing with in order to understand the miasms. Let's see what miasms Hahnemann referred to and how he defined them in *Chronic Diseases*. He talked about acute miasms and the smallpox vaccination. He says in a footnote:

CD We may justly ask: Is there in any probability any miasma in the world, which, when it has infected from without, does not first make the whole organism sick before the signs of it externally manifest themselves? We can only answer this questions with, *no*, there is none (1997, Vol. 1, pp. 33)!

The latter is also expressed in Aphorisms 201 to 202. Also in *Chronic Diseases*, Hahnemann discussed this in the same fashion when he described a person becoming infected with anthrax or other acute illnesses:

> **CD** The same is the case, not to mention several other acute miasms, also when the skin of man is contaminated with the blood of cattle affected with anthrax. If, as is frequently the case, the anthrax has infected and caught on, all removal of skin is in vain; the black or gangrenous blister, nearly always fatal, nevertheless, always comes out four or five days later (usually in the affected spot); *i.e.*, as soon as the whole living organism has transformed itself to this terrible disease. ... From the progress of all these miasmatic diseases we may plainly see that, after the contagion from without, the malady connected with it in the interiors of the whole man must be developed; *i.e.*, the whole interior man must first have become thoroughly sick of smallpox, measles or scarlet fever, before these various eruptions may appear on the skin (Ibid, p. 33-34).

In modern times we refer to this as the *incubation* period, but often the exterior relief of the internal generalized disease (Aphorisms 201-202) is still treated in allopathy as if it were a localized disease, that is, often by suppressing the symptoms. In *Chronic Diseases*, Hahnemann says further:

> **CD** It is just so with the infection of half-acute miasms without eruptions. Among many persons bitten by a mad dog ... only a few are infected ... often, as I myself have observed, only one out of twenty or thirty persons bitten. The others, even if ever so badly mangled by the mad dog, usually all recover, even if they are not treated by a physician or surgeon. [And allopaths give those painful shots if the virus is found in the dog!] But with whomsoever the poison acts, it has taken effect in the moment when the person was bitten, and the poison has then communicated itself to the nearest nerves and, therefore, without contradiction, to the whole system of the nerves, and as soon as the malady has developed in the whole organism (for this development and completion of the disease nature requires at least several days, often many weeks), the madness breaks out as an acute, quickly fatal disease. ... even immediate excision and amputation of the infected part does not protect from the progression of the disease within ... (Ibid, p. 34).

The hydrophobia miasm is termed "half acute" because it takes a long time for this miasm to completely develop in the system before the symptoms manifest, although once these symptoms manifest, the patient suffers as though from an acute disease.

The acute miasms of whooping cough, smallpox, measles, etc. have been termed "fixed miasms" by Hahnemann, because whenever these diseases occur, they show the same clinical features.

—

Contrary to the case of chronic miasms, there is hope for a more favorable outcome with acute ones—unless the patient is overcome by the acute disease. As Hahnemann writes in *Chronic Diseases*:

> **CD** For all these *acute* miasmatic diseases the human constitution possesses that process [he is referring to the VF and what allopathy would now call the "immune system"] which, as a rule, is so beneficent: to wipe them out (*i.e.*, the specific fever together with the specific eruption) in the course of from two to three weeks, and of itself to extinguish them again, through a kind of decision (*crisis*), from the organism [reaction of the VF], so that man then is wont to be entirely healed of them and, indeed, in a short time, unless he be killed by them (Ibid, p. 35).

In the case of acute diseases, there are two other options apart from those suggested in the previous paragraph. The acute disease could now become a chronic illness, stronger than the previous chronic natural disease or the newly formed chronic disease could join forces with the old chronic disease and form a complex disease, more difficult to treat. Hahnemann continues:

> **CD** In the chronic miasmatic diseases nature observes *the same course* with respect to the mode of contagion and the antecedent formation of the internal disease, before the external declarative symptoms of its internal completion manifests itself on the surface of the body; but then that great remarkable difference from the acute diseases shows itself, that in the chronic miasmata the entire internal disease, as we have mentioned before, remains in the organism during the whole life, yea, it increases with every year, if it is not exterminated and thoroughly cured *by art* [homeopathy] (Ibid, p. 35).

Thus, the homeopath must recognize the importance of acknowledging and assessing true *chronic* miasmatic states as they can *never* be cured by the constitution, not by the best lifestyle, nor by diet, in spite of what macrobiotic or vegetarian adherents claim! The homeopath must also understand that chronic miasmatic states do not exist in pure form, that is, solely on the physical, the mental, or the emotional level. Life is always a mixture. All three planes are always more or less affected. Moreover, the person is usually affected by more than one miasmatic state; it is the homeopath's task to determine what constitutes the patient's active miasmatic state versus the dormant/latent one(s) at the moment of consultation.

The Basic Chronic Miasms

I have studied the *Organon* many times and try to stay strictly within the guidelines Hahnemann laid down, as I have never been disappointed by them. To those who consider the *Organon* a "dusty old bible," I have two points to make: show me one aphorism that is incorrect and, secondly, what have you (or anyone else for that matter) discovered that could be the basis for a 7th edition of the *Organon?* No matter what anyone claims, no one in modern times has been able to add anything that was not already tried by Hahnemann. And that's simply because Hahnemann completed this science during his own lifetime. I am not referring to neo-guru homeopaths who trample on basic homeopathic laws in order to make their "new artistic theory" acceptable. They suspend true Hahnemannian homeopathy with theories full of imagination, projection, and, as some call it, intuition. Nowadays the homeopath is overwhelmed by so many "different" miasms that he needs to ask the basic question: "How many different miasms are really possible?" I went to the source, the *Organon,* and studied carefully the parts where Hahnemann discusses miasms.

In **Aphorism 74**, Hahnemann starts talking about the miasms. This aphorism provided me with new insight and the true definition of the miasms and led me to correct some inaccurate conclusions I had drawn in the past. In this aphorism, Hahnemann talks about how chronic diseases get artificially created by allopathic treatment, by the prolonged use of violent, heroic drugs, etc. (iatrogenic diseases). Hahnemann says that all these measures:

> **A 74** ... relentlessly weaken the vital force and, if they do not completely exhaust it, progressively untune it, each in its own characteristic way, to such an extent that it has to bring about a *revolution* in the organism to maintain life against these hostile and destructive attacks (emphasis added).

So far what Hahnemann is saying is that the VF, being attacked and mistuned so relentlessly, creates a *defense* mechanism (he calls it a revolution) in order to survive these hostile attacks. In the next paragraph of this aphorism, Hahnemann tells us clearly that there are only *three major chronic miasms,* simply because there are only *three major defense mechanisms in any organism, starting with the individual cell.* All other modern miasms are thus pseudo-miasms or mixed miasms! Miasms are defensive responses of the cell. Let's consider what Hahnemann says:

> **A 74** ... It [the cell] has to *inhibit or exaggerate* the excitability or sensitivity of a part of the organism, *dilate or contract, soften or harden,* or even completely *destroy* certain parts, and bring about internal or external lesions (internally or externally maiming the body) in order to protect the organism against complete destruction of life from the ever renewed hostile attacks of such ruinous forces (emphasis added).

In this same aphorism, speaking of iatrogenic diseases, he cites especially bloodletting and the starvation diet as the two major ruinous forces that destroyed the organism in his time. Unfortunately we have many more iatrogenic diseases today.

Looking further at Aphorism 74, we see that Hahnemann describes three possible different defense mechanisms:

1. Inhibition or deprivation (loss of function) or exaggeration of excitability (which translates into irritation or acute inflammation) or sensitivity (hypersensitivity) of a part of the organism. This is called *psora, a physiological defense*: it shuts down or increases the organism's reactivity. In Traditional Chinese Medicine (TCM), this would be called a general Qi deficiency.

2. Dilatation (cysts) or contraction, softening (relaxed tendons and ligaments leading to prolapse of the organs or collapse in general) or hardening (induration). This represents *sycosis or constructive defense*. According to Hahnemann, there are two sycotic forms: one of *over*-construction (induration, hardening, contraction), one of *under*-construction (collapse, dilatation, softening, relaxing). In TCM, the latter would be called Yang Excess Qi.

3. Complete destruction is expressed through the *syphilitic miasm* (*destructive defense*). In TCM, it would be called Yin Excess Qi.

According to this definition, only the latter two miasms bring structural changes whereas psora produces only physiological changes. Thus, a living being has only three defense types. As a defensive response to invasion of a microorganism, every cell will inflame, indurate, or be destroyed in an attempt to maintain the well-being of the person as a whole!

Psora: First Line of Defense

The *first line of defense* of a cell is *inflammation*, a protective response which is preceded by irritation and increased sensitivity: rubor, calor, dolor, and then finally loss of function. All these changes are observed in the physiological defense of any cell. The cell's response starts with hypoxia and ischemia, creating an environment unsuitable to microorganisms where the oxygen and blood supply is cut off. The sole aim of this defense mechanism is to kill the microorganism by temporarily changing the biochemistry within the cell or neighboring tissue. So every cell at first defends itself by a process of inflammation or hypersensitivity or irritation but eventually progresses to loss of function or at least hypo-function. Therefore all diseases which fall into inflammatory stages due to chemical, biochemical, or physiological changes, hypo-nutrition, and malabsorption are *psoric diseases*. *No structural* changes are noted as yet!

This means that the psoric diseases will be all the *acute "itis"* diseases (please note that this is a correction to what I wrote in *Hahnemann Revisited*) as well as dermatitis, eczema, pharyngitis, and functional disturbances of the nervous system such as anxiety neurosis, vertigo, and epilepsy—the latter being a grafting of the syphilitic miasm on the psoric. Psoric diseases are easily seen in the gastrointestinal tract, the genitourinary tract, and the respiratory tract. They include all functional derangements as well as hyper- and hypo-sensitivity. Whenever there is much anxiety (about health, about being unable to accomplish what they want to do, about not being able to carry out their plans), apprehension, irritability, lack of confidence or inhibition (timidity), it is psora. With heart symptoms, for example, there is always anxiety about an imminent attack or a fit on the part of the patient: he constantly checks his pulse. Grief and sorrow are two of the main emotions that awaken the psoric miasm. The psoric person will weep often and is relieved from it. Certainly, a psoric patient demands much attention from his physician.

Hypersensitivity and *reactivity*, in response to environmental stimuli, are hallmarks of the psoric miasm. What happens in hypersensitivity? The system gears itself towards restoring a healthy balance through immediate, adequate mobilization of the natural defenses at its disposal, seeking a return to normalcy. A clear example is how *simple* inflammatory processes resolve rapidly without suppuration and residue, leaving no troublesome effects. Psora is all about a normal inflammatory process. In this way, the troublesome effects are restricted to the level of the skin and appendages and the level of the mind (theorizing, making plans, abundance of ideas, irritability, etc.).

Eruptions are manifestations of *primary* psora. When these expressions are suppressed, there is a progressive internalization of the trouble towards more vital organs (to the lungs in the first place, according to TCM; note the known progression from eczema to asthma!) and this creates *secondary* psoric expressions, functional changes, but still with minimal or no structural alterations, thus the symptoms are reversible.

Let's list some examples of psora, with many more to be found in Volume I of *Chronic Diseases* (Ibid, pp. 45-47; pp. 51-77):

- Labile hypertension under stress and "white coat syndrome"

- Deficiencies (minerals, enzymes, vitamins, salts) that require replacement therapy

- Perspiration on the head, in the evening after going to sleep

- Frequent inflammation of the eyes

- Frequent cramps in the calves

- Frequent attacks of dyspnea

- Many scales on the scalp

- Dryness of mucosa

- Functional derangements

- Very pale tongue

- Aversion to meat

- Malabsorption, malnutrition

- Impotency

- Hypersensitive reactions to vaccinations.

That psora is always the first line of defense is easily seen in the portraits of homeopathic remedies according to the provings, see the example of *Lachesis* in Chapter 7. The organism, no matter how negative the core delusion, will always try *first* to find constructive or positive compensations. Only when this does not work will the compensations change to exaggeration (sycosis) or destruction (syphilis) as seen in the remedy provings according to Hahnemann.

It is wise of us to use some *synonyms* that express what psora really stands for. We can go through the following list to see if it corresponds to the patient's expressions and symptoms:

Synonyms or Expressions of the Psoric Miasm

Inflammation, lack of (in the sense of *less*), *deficiency*, insufficiency, inhibition or being tied down, hypersensitive, needing and giving support, affection and protection, deprivation-weakness-inferiority complex, timidity, fault-finding, coldness, slowness, passivity, stagnation, immobility, non-productive, non-action, mulling it over, temperate, introvert, denial, stasis, laziness, motionless, postponing, dependence, attachment, subservience, vulnerability, helplessness, oversensitive to odors, never satisfied, lacking power of assimilation, desire to rest, inability to relax, desire to lie down, lack of concentration, unable to finish tasks because of lack of stamina, indulgent, making plans.

When the individual is inhibited, his modes of expressions are reduced, he is poorly nourished, and he becomes debilitated. All the organs and their cells produce an insufficiency, reflected in physiological weakness and limited possibilities. The psoric person demands pity and obtains it as if it were something made expressly for him. It is this characteristic that reflects his egotism as he focuses on his ailments and pesters everyone around him with trifles): a possessive, enduring anxiety. To compensate for this deficiency, either excess (sycosis) or perversion (syphilis) will result. So psora is the *basic* condition of all human pathology.

Sycosis: Second Line of Defense

When bacteria try to invade, and the "irritation" continues, it turns into *chronic* inflammation. The acute inflammation or psoric expression has shifted to a chronic inflammatory reaction due to the cell's unsuccessful response that was aimed at creating circumstances impenetrable to the microorganisms. The cells are obliged to shift to another line of defense, a *structural* or morphological defense. This is called sycosis and can be of *two different types*:

1. The first form of sycosis is *over-construction*. The cells say, "I've built an impenetrable wall around me (induration or thickening) so that I am better protected." This is just like wearing a shoe that is too narrow: first you get irritation and inflammation (psora), then, if it continues, a corn or bunion develops (induration or sycosis), and if the situation continues an ulcer forms (syphilitic). Induration is *excessive fibrin*. Contraction of tissues is caused by *excess elastine*. In excessive cell multiplication, one cell divides into many, giving rise to tumors, growths, thickening, and accumulation which corresponds to sycotic excess or over-construction. The sycotic person will also build a wall around himself emotionally to protect himself: *Natrum muriaticum* is a good example of that. He will also use other sycotic expressions such as lying or boasting to build an excessive persona.

2. Besides over-construction, sycosis also can exhibit *under-construction*. Hahnemann refers to this in Aphorism 74 as "dilatation (caused by lack of fibrin) and relaxation (caused by lack of elastine)."

It is interesting that the homeopath can find under- and over-construction expressed in the king of anti-sycotic remedies, *Thuja*. We find the delusions: *appearance of building stones* (over-construction) and *body is made of glass, body is brittle* (under-construction). Slow recovery and growing speed of pathology are hallmarks of the sycotic miasm.

Examples of Sycotic Excess or Over-Construction

Obesity (over-accumulation of fat); warts or skin tags (over-accumulation of skin); edema (excess accumulation of water in ascites in liver cancer, hydrothorax in heart deficiency, vesicles, bullae, and painful menstrual irregularities with

PMS and swelling of breasts); fibroids; atherosclerosis (excessive fibrin); hypertension, resulting from damage to the vascular bed of the kidneys and salt and water retention; induration (excess accumulation of fibrin as in styes); hyperlipedemia (excess accumulation of fat) and hypercholesterolemia; darkening of skin and moles, liver spots, freckles and naevus: excess accumulation of melanocytes due to imbalance of adrenal cortical hormone production; keloids; and renal stones. Excessive leucocytosis or leukemia is sycotic. Hypertrophies; hyperplasia of cervical mucosa; ketosis; gout (excessive uric acid crystals, which become worse with over-indulgence in food or wine); and constriction, stenosis, and strictures (excess elastine). Thick, rigid, and heavy nails.

Other examples of excess generation: gallstones and kidney stones; deposition of calcium in normal tissues; tartar on teeth; salivary gland calculus; pigmentation of skin, brown spots, liver spots; osteophytes, spurs, osteomas; hemangiomas, varicose veins, and hemorrhoids; cysts; polyps; endometriosis; corns; callus; ringworm, and hirsutism (abnormal hair growth whether localized or generalized).

Sycotic discharges are typically acrid, thick, and greenish-yellow, with a briny odor. Perspiration stains yellow. Non-specific urethritis (NSU) and Reiter's syndrome (urethritis, arthritis, and uveitis) are due to chronic inflammation where suppression has taken place. Rheumatoid Arthritis is also sycotic. Also fibromyalgia (chronic fibrositis in large muscles) is an expression of rheumatic constitutions which tend to be worse in cold damp weather and from rest. All *chronic "itis"* expressions are sycotic. A great example is Pelvic Inflammatory Disease, as are all inflammatory diseases of the female genital tract, which can be traced to the sycotic taint.

What about diabetes? If it is the result of an inflammation of the Islets of Langerhans or impaired blood flow due to constriction of vessels, then the psoric miasm is indicated. If the diabetes is due to atherosclerosis, then sycosis is implicated and may be accompanied by weight gain (which can be corrected by dietary changes), Type II diabetes, or Non-Insulin Dependent Diabetes. If there is cellular destruction, then the syphilitic miasm is at work (as in juvenile and insulin-dependent diabetes: Type I diabetes).

Examples of Sycotic Under-Construction

Hypo-pigmentation (not vitiligo, which is syphilitic in nature and melanocytes are destroyed) and tinea versicolor (lack of melanin). Dwarfism (excess height and insufficient height are both sycotic). *Hypo-function* of all organs: hypothyroid, hypotension, of kidneys, etc. and *prolapse* (lack of elastine) are sycotic.

Other sycotic examples include varicose veins; prolapsed uterus, hemorrhoids or piles; ptosis of viscera; mitral valve prolapse (MVP); relaxed muscles and tendons with recurrent spraining; osteoporosis (progressive decrease in density); anemia if caused by lack of iron; and alopecia areata.

Sycosis exhibits fear, fright, insecurity with love for life (sometimes to the extreme expressed in *carpe diem* or "seize the day"), and fear of death. In sycosis there is usually one outspoken fear at a time (i.e., fear of dying), in psora many anxieties exist at the same time. If you send a sycotic and a psoric person into a dark building, the psoric will have many anxieties: "Will someone hurt me? What if there is a dog to bite me? Will something fall on me?" "Am I going to be robbed?" In other words, many thoughts go through his mind (*theorizing*). The sycotic person might just fear one thing but since he is a boaster he may say, "I'm not afraid, but I have no time to go in now," in other words he will find an excuse! He will hide one aspect of his being, often sexual in nature.

Sycosis also deals with *sexuality*, either excess or too little. Increased sexual desires are sycotic: nymphomania, erotomania, masturbation, and womanizing (*Medorrhinum, Lycopodium, Apis*). Only when perversion (incest, sado-masochism) sets in does the compensation become syphilitic. An example of a luetic sexual remedy is *Cantharis* who above all wants to satisfy himself; the material substance was used by the Marquis de Sade in his sexual addiction. *Cantharis* also has that violent, burning, stinging sensation. It creates an excessive urge that the person is not able to control, a syphilitic expression. Furthermore, in sycosis we find cunning, hiding, deceitfulness, jealousy, secretiveness, and boasting. His suspicion is extreme to the point where he constantly has to go back and check on himself: "Did I lock the door?" This is expressed by the rubric: *Forgotten, something; feels constantly as if he had forgotten* (*Causticum* and *Iodum* are the main remedies).

Synonyms or Expressions of the Sycotic Miasm

Proliferation, induration, neo-formations, hyperplasia; instable, capricious, changeable, inconsistent (formerly called the tubercular miasm!), ostentatious, explosive, *excessive*; escapism, flight, hiding, volubility, over-production, exuberance, foolishness; exploiting, ambitious, presumptuous, impertinent, extravert, flamboyant, eloquent; self-condemnation, fixed ideas (delusions), deposits, rapid progression, corrosive discharges, competitive, and passionate.

Syphilitic Miasm: Third Line of Cellular Defense or Destruction

Among the three basic chronic miasms, the syphilitic is the easiest to cure as long as it is not complicated with psora or sycosis.

There are two destructive types:

• Autoimmune disorders (rheumatoid arthritis, Hashimoto's disease, Crohn's disease, colitis ulcerosa, etc.) where the body kills itself through formation of antibodies against its own cells (*apolysis*).

• The other type is *necrosis*: the body tries to cut off a particular part and wall it off as dead tissue (heart infarct, gangrene).

There are two distinctly different classes of syphilitic remedies. Some, such as *Aurum muriaticum*, kill themselves because they are driven by their core delusion! Others, such as *Mercurius, Anacardium, Alumina, Syphilinum, Tarentula*, and *Hyoscyamus*, kill others! And they may kill without much apparent provocation and without any fear for consequences: to obtain power or money, to escape from domination (*Anacardium, Alumina*), to bind the attention of loved ones to themselves (*Hyoscyamus*), etc.

The syphilitic miasm means that the person "has totally lost control over their actions", as seen in the rubrics: *Out of control* and *thoughts, control of thoughts lost*. They don't care what happens to their own or to others' lives, they show no remorse, are disobedient, and lie. They lack moral feeling! The syphilitic miasm is also expressed in *anguish* and *despair with giving up all hope*.

Examples of Syphilitic Diseases

Disfigurement, gangrene, ulcerations, bleeding, deep bleeding cracks, ozaena, azoospermia, cataract, caries of cartilage, cleft palate, blindness, deafness, renal failure, paralysis, heart infarct, lung fibrosis, emphysema, Parkinson's disease, multiple sclerosis, ALS, Alzheimer's disease, etc.

What About Alcoholism?

It can start as social drinking in which people drink to feel less inhibited in public (psora). Then they get hooked on it and start drinking on the sly (e.g., drinking mother tinctures because of the alcohol content) and hide this drinking from their loved ones (sycosis). Ultimately drinking becomes a necessity for them, destroying themselves and their family (syphilitic).

Synonyms or Expressions of the Syphilitic Miasm

*Destruction from the **onset** of the disease*, dysplasia, burning, bleeding, agenesis of organs, deformation, *sudden* ulceration with bleeding, loss of sensory senses, fissures, cracks, decay, gangrene, atrophy, underdevelopment of organs (infantile), structural bone changes, fighting, out of control (uncontrolled behavior, growth, etc.), aggressiveness toward others, self-degeneration, violence, passion, *perversion*, unrepentant, mutilation, subduing, dominating others, incest, forgetful about what they say or read, nocturnal aggravation, introvert, and overwhelmed.

Miasms: A Predisposed, Mandatory, Fixed Response Pattern

If there are only three defense mechanisms for the cell, then there are only three for the human being: What is true for the cell is true for the whole organism. What does this mean? Whatever constitutional miasm you received from your parents will be your automatic, predisposed, fixed response pattern (Carl Jung). When the homeopath determines the patient's predominant miasmatic state, he can predict what kind of diseases this patient will suffer from. When psoric constitutions fall ill, they will fight back with physiological defenses (remedies like *Sulphur, Nux vomica, Calcarea carbonica, Belladonna*, etc.). The sycotic constitution will react either with over- or under-construction. Therefore, the great sycotic remedies pass very quickly from psoric compensations to sycotic ones. Strongly syphilitic remedies, such as *Mercurius, Fluoricum acidum, Alumina*, etc., move rapidly and easily from psora straight to syphilis. In such cases, a simple stomach or duodenal inflammation leads to *immediate* ulceration with bleeding and rupture.

Most diseases with deep-seated pathology are tri-miasmatic. Psoriasis is an example: excessive proliferation of ectoderm with excessive scaling in dermis (psora and sycosis). When there are cracks and bleeding, it becomes syphilitic. Another example is the fish scale eruption (ichtyosis), which has the dryness of psora, the squamous character of the syphilitic eruption, and the moles and warts of sycosis.

The Acceleration of the Miasmatic Cycle in Modern Times

Over time most diseases follow the same pattern: *Inflammation > Growth > Destruction*. When an illness is not treated homeopathically or when it is treated with suppressive allopathic measures, the patient's illness slides from psoric to sycotic to syphilitic means of compensation.

Sulphur (like *Calcarea carbonica, Lycopodium, Silicea*, etc.) is a tri-miasmatic remedy: normally in childhood this person is psoric with eczema and rashes. Around the age of 24, *Sulphur* becomes sycotic and starts using alcohol and drugs; he starts boasting, becomes loquacious, and sexual thoughts intrude on his mind. Still later *Sulphur* becomes the burnt-out hermit (syphilitic). Nowadays, with all the suppressive allopathic medications and vaccinations, we push youngsters into a sycotic state even earlier than 50 years ago. Look at the obesity and diabetes epidemics that are starting at a very early age in the United States (sycosis due to dietary mistakes). Homeopathic intervention can stop this rapid downward spiral from one miasmatic state to the next.

There is a condition called Non-Alcoholic Steato Hepatitis (NASH), which entails fatty degeneration of the liver with progression to cirrhosis. NASH is mainly associated with obesity (70 to 100 percent of the cases) and diabetes. This is often seen with diabetic patients, but NASH is now seen in children! I wonder how much the present explosion of vaccines contributes to this condition as well. Allopathy claims that "just because you are overweight it does not mean you have diabetes. You need to have the gene for it." But allopathy can't predict whether you will become diabetic or not. Homeopaths understand this better. The "gene" is the sycotic or syphilitic miasm. If one of these two is predominant, the patient will pass from obesity to diabetes type I or II.

The current list for newborns of 22 vaccinations in the first two years of life and the reckless prescription of antibiotics are two major causes pushing our children to a sycotic state at an early age. Add to this the lack of prenatal parental miasmatic treatment leading to a transfer of these miasmatic states to their children at birth. The explosion of ADD, OCD, ASD, as well as countless other challenged children is the unfortunate proof of this theory.

One Golden Prescribing Tip

If the case and the chief complaint (CC) are predominantly syphilitic, for example, then to find the simillimum the homeopath takes only the syphilitic rubrics of the case into account! The same is true for the other miasms!

Determining the Miasmatic State

Why are children within one family so different? They have the same parents and yet sometimes it appears that a child "belongs to another family." Sometimes in a neurotic family, one child reacts with hysteria (sycosis), another with a compulsion disorder (sycosis), the third one with a psychosis (luetic), and the fourth apparently not at all? This is not an **elective** "choice of neurosis."

First of all, the gender determines the predominant miasm. The miasm usually crosses gender: for a boy, look at his mother's history. For a girl, look first at the father's history. Of course, when there are three boys, we can always clearly see which boy received his father's or mother's miasm.

Secondly, as seen in TCM, much depends on the physical, mental, and emotional state of the parents at the *moment* of conception; on the parents' *ages*; and of course on *what happened* during the pregnancy (the 10 Intrauterine questions; see Chap. 13). The all important Kidney Yin Qi will be less (in amount or in quality) if parents are in distress, older, overworked, etc.

A tennis friend of mine is a clear example of this. He has three children, the youngest being 6 years old, the older ones 9 and 11. He told me that his youngest son broke his femur in a simple fall, that he had already broken his humerus at age one, and that he also suffered from a hearing defect. These are all expressions of a deficient Kidney Essence. In fact, I did not have to ask if this was the youngest child. The two older children did not suffer at all from these problems so the age of parents at conception (father was 47; mother was 43) was past the ideal moment to conceive a child. In addition, the mother was in a *Sepia* state, which contributed to these "syphilitic" defects in the youngest child!

To determine the miasmatic state, first *observe* the patient! Each individual has a different physical make-up; each carries the stigma of his inherited defects, faults of nutrition, lifestyle, and illness—often clearly visible to our eyes. These stigmas (one or more of the miasms) will be reflected in each human being due to the multiple pathological inheritances we all carry within ourselves. The man who presents as shy, observing, timid, introspective, who walks slowly and whose actions reveal a passive nature has the visiting card of a psoric person. The person who walks with her midriff exposed; rings in her nose, belly button, and lips; has a body full of tattoos; sways as she walks; and is always in a hurry has a predominating sycotic quality. And the syphilitic person who always has an ill-looking, somber expression; fish eyes that undress you from top to bottom; always in a morose, fretful, and peevish mood; despises everyone; and is always ready to be aggressive and strike out (as if he *is engaged in lawsuits*) carries the syphilitic miasm.

The homeopath must always keep in mind that all three miasms will most likely be manifested at some point in an individual. Even when his attitude, manners, and appearance correspond *mainly* to one of these miasmatic traits, the person will still exhibit certain traits and some manifestations of the other two miasms, although at each stage of his life, one of the three will predominate, and you may only catch a slight glimpse of the other miasmatic traits.

Although psora is the dominant miasm, the homeopath must remember that there will be innumerable psoric types that will all contain a taint of the other two miasms in differing degrees, on a scale of 1 to 100, 1 being the purely psoric miasm, 100 the most miasmatically-mixed patient.

To one who wants to be a true homeopath, the enormous utility, indeed indispensability of the knowledge of the miasmatic modulations in every human being is self-evident. Classifying all the individual's expressions (symptoms) in accordance with the characteristics of each miasm is a must in order to understand how these miasms hamper and deform his individuality. This certainly provides the best method for deducing the patient's prognosis. Only through *prenatal* homeopathic miasmatic treatment can the homeopath succeed in treating the child at the same time as the mother, a benefit that has been bestowed on homeopathy more than on any other modality. TCM and allopathy have to treat the pregnant mother with utmost care and suspend many of their regular interventions. With prenatal homeopathic care, the eugenic benefits of truly homeopathic treatment throughout successive generations would become clear. Only by using constitutionally prescribed medicines, in the true Hahnemannian fashion, can the genuine physician effectively promote eugenics or true genetic therapy. Alas, we are still far from achieving this because of continued allopathic suppression and, let's face it, because of inadequate homeopathic practice worldwide.

A good eugenic formula should not be restricted to chromosomal factors or mutational possibilities as defined in allopathy. These are just convenient labels. The real formula should be deduced from dynamic elements: psychic, spiritual, sensorial, even telluric (environment-related) ones.

Responsible Procreation

All our actions in life have been predetermined by the dominant miasmatic state produced by our parents, grandparents, etc. It is therefore imperative for the present generation to start taking responsibility (and I address my words first to the homeopathic world, since we have the key to the door) and undergo miasmatic treatment before procreation. All our actions and words, our mental make-up and thoughts, and our degree of intelligence depend on a clean miasmatic slate. Let's take a look at an example of how the different dominant miasmatic states react to a certain situation.

Let's say the psoric person is caught in a fire on the 13th floor of a building, as was the case in the horrible events of 9/11. First, such a person will be overwhelmed, paralyzed; then he will start thinking what to do, mulling things over, though it is always difficult for him to force his body into movement. He will

—

seek an exit, call for help, pray to God to rescue him, promise to do good deeds when he gets out of this situation, or trust that someone will come to help him. You don't need to tell him, "Stay put." He does. Rather we need to remind him to *act* after debating what to do.

The sycotic person is always *hasty*, in a hurry, even in his decisions. He is prompt and, without thinking, acts on his first impulse. He might go right through the flames because the exit is behind them; he might jump out of the window without thinking of the consequences, again just acting on first impulse. He will forget everything, even his child next to him. The extravert sycotic person always acts first, then thinks.

The syphilitic individual will fall into a state of terror, which prompts him to do destructive things. It makes him desperate and even though he knows he will die if he jumps, he still will do it. Or he might kill himself and his beloved "to spare her the suffering." This may look like an act of benevolence, but it really is a reflection of his bottled-up syphilitic aggression.

Each of these individuals has acted according to his miasmatic burden: he has been *forced*, by these hereditary factors, to act this way. Jung called this the "fixed, mandatory inherited response pattern." No one has the right to condemn someone because they are victims of "guilty" parents. The psoric person may go through life burdened by his complaints and impotence. The sycotic person may be the subject of scandal and even responsible for crimes committed for the thrill. The syphilitic person can be the true criminal, distrusted by everyone, including himself. Yet the homeopath must have empathy for all these patients. Only through well-selected homeopathic remedies and good case management can the homeopath avert such situations in the first place. The homeopath, knowing that a patient's miasmatic burden will influence their children, should counsel prospective parents to pursue homeopathic treatment—for both partners—before thinking of having a child. They are responsible for bringing healthy children into the world.

Applying the Miasmatic Concept in Practice

1. Take a complete personal history: from day one on up to the moment of consultation, indicating where suppressive therapies took place. Include the family history and remember that there is frequently transference to the opposite gender.

2. From the onset of life, try to identify the predominant miasm, the latent miasm, and secondary miasmatic states. A good timeline with precise dates is necessary. A remedy is palliative if we don't see miasmatic improvement.

Hering's Set of Observations can help the homeopath assess improvement and determine whether mere palliation or actual changes in the miasmatic state have occurred with the remedy.

3. Correlate the indicated layer remedy with the miasm expressed in the CC. This miasmatic knowledge will be used to differentiate between remedies, that is, if the CC is syphilitic, the simillimum should be the strongest syphilitic remedy among those that are close at the end of the investigation.

Always keep in mind that miasmatic progression and disease progression run parallel; hence Hering's Set of Observations. Miasmatic improvement must be clinically observed in tandem with the process of healing.

Denoting Miasmatic Tendencies of Clinical Expressions

I will give some examples that reflect the three different miasmatic expressions. I must emphasize that a single symptom cannot represent the whole state (as the homeopath should know from reading the footnote of **Aphorism 7**) and that a single miasmatic expression will *not* indicate the whole dominant miasmatic condition of the patient; *only* the totality will count. But it is the analysis of all these separate symptoms that will give the homeopath the whole picture. So far no good homeopathic book has been written that correctly translates our rubrics into miasmatic expressions. It is not my goal in this book to do so, as that is a huge work which I will hope to address in a future book. The few books and the few computer programs that reflect this miasmatic division are either based on guesswork or inaccurate information. It will be a great gift to homeopathy when each remedy is given a miasmatic denotation in all its true proving expressions. Only then can such findings withstand close scrutiny; the homeopath will be able to see why a particular remedy is X% psoric, Y% sycotic, and Z% syphilitic.

In the following examples, predominant psora will be indicated with capital "P," predominant sycosis with "S," and predominant syphilis with "L" (luetic). If an expression is secondary (i.e., not as strong as the primary miasmatic influence but strong enough to change its characteristics somewhat), it is denoted with a lowercase letter. For example, the rubric expressing predominant psora and secondary syphilis is denoted as "P/l." It is beyond the scope of this book to elaborate with many examples, but I trust that the few examples I can provide in this chapter will clarify and support the miasmatic theory.

We must emphasize again that a single symptom does not represent the whole (see footnote of Aphorism 7) and that a single miasmatic expression will NOT denote the whole miasmatic dominant condition of the patient; only the totality will count. But it is the analysis of all these separate symptoms that will give us the whole picture.

—

Psoric Symptoms	Sycotic Symptoms	Syphilitic Symptoms
Constipation	Diarrhea	Dysentery
Slow peristalsis	Accelerated	Spasm
Bradycardia	Tachycardia	Arrhythmia
Dry mucosa	Increased secretion	Ulceration, fistula
Anxiety	Fear	Panic/Terror/Anguish
Religious	Fanatic	Agnostic
Pain: Lame, bruised	Pain: Lancinating, stitching, stabbing, electrical, spastic, prickling	Pain: Burning, tearing, ulcerating
Thin/sinewy	Obese	Emaciated
Timidity	Audacity	Recklessness
Loves others	Loves the self	Loves no one
Irritation	Induration	Destruction
Timidity	Lack of confidence (P/s)	Incapacity
Weariness of life	Loathing of life	Suicidal disposition
Immobilized when confronted with fear or danger	Flight; Startled	Fight
Annoyed/Irritated	Anger (Ire)	Rage/Fury
Sadness	Grief	Depression
Stuck	Hurry	Delirious
Absorbed	Delusion	Delirium
Introverted when disappointed	Talks to others when disappointed	Collapses from disappointment
Joy	Hysteria/Mirth	Exhilaration
Complaining	Moaning	Lamenting
Lasciviousness (S/p)	Shameless	Lewdness
Frivolity (S/p)	Libertinism	Want of moral feeling
White/yellow discharges	Yellow/green discharges	Bloody/red/necrotic discharges

Let's elaborate on some of the examples listed above.

Degrees of Anxiety

Anxiety takes on diverse forms and expressions. For example, a person can have anxiety about going insane, anxiety others will observe his apprehension, anxiety of suffering misfortune, anxiety about trifles, anxiety with fear of death, anxiety about anticipating an event, anxiety about health. All these symptoms are part of the patient's elaboration of psoric anxiety. In the psoric person, we always see many anxieties expressed at the same time. He feels his pulse, checks his blood pressure, and wants the doctor to conduct tests. If psora dominates, fear does not attain its full extent but remains as anxiety, which is the antechamber or forerunner of fear. If the anxieties increase, the person usually starts concentrating on one topic and becomes truly fearful.

Fear is sycotic, and the patient's emotional state is predominated by it. An example is *Chelidonium's* fear that his health is ruined. Fears that become outspoken turn into delusions or fixed ideas (*Chelidonium* has the same delusion). This permanency and intensity denotes sycosis. The person is dominated by this emotion. But he desperately tries to compensate for his fear or delusion and does not entirely lose control over his actions.

When fear overwhelms the patient, it becomes **anguish**—a permanent state that paralyzes the patient. Anguish tends to be a syphilitic expression. He becomes stuck, hopeless, and gives up. He has lost control over his life and is unable to proceed further. He basically has the attitude that nothing can be done, and refuses medicine. A perfect example is *Aconite* who is convinced he will die at a specific time and that nothing can be done. Anguish may be accompanied by suicidal thoughts, as seen, for example, in patients needing *Hepar sulph*. When anguish accompanies anger (L/s), think of *Platina*. Anguish with colic (L/s) may call for *Coffea*. Anguish after hearing horrible things (L/p) may indicate *Calcarea carbonica*. And when *Phosphoric acid* experiences anguish, they must lie down (L/p). Anguish with palpitations (L/s) can indicate *Arsenicum* and *Phosphorus*.

Religious Expressions

For the psoric person, a belief in God stands for unending desire for absolute protection, to be free of pain and suffering. For example, *Calcarea carbonica* is listed in the rubrics: *religious, wants to read the Bible all day* (pure psora) and *religious affections about metaphysical concerns* (pure psora). *Platina* has a purely psoric expression: *wants to do penance*.

Sycotic patients, however, may display religious fanaticism and mania, for example, *Veratrum album* and *Sulphur*. In patients needing *Hyoscyamus*, we see: *talking of religious subjects* (pure sycosis). A syphilitic patient may be an agnostic (*Lachesis*).

Expressions About the Desire to Live

Psoric patients experience the symptom **weariness of life**, which is a feeling like being tired after a long walk. For example, if a *Phosphorus* constitution becomes extremely exhausted, they can transition into a state requiring *Phosphoric acid*, which is graded a 2 for the symptom: *weariness of life*. The person can't move forward. Everything in life feels heavy, everything is a chore, and the person does not experience joy; every aspect is cumbersome (pure psora).

Sycotic patients take weariness of life a step further and experience the symptom **loathing of life**, which is a lack of enthusiasm for life, indifference to life (e.g., *Natrum muriaticum, Staphysagria, Sepia*). With *loathing of life*, the patient feels life has no meaning (a spiritual disease). The person is indifferent to pleasurable things and lacks *joie de vivre*.

Moving beyond loathing for life, the syphilitic patient may develop **persistent thoughts about death** and can even derive pleasure from having suicidal thoughts (*Aurum* is purely luetic; L). The rubric, *persistent thoughts of suicide but lacks courage* (*Nux vomica, China*), is a luetic and psoric expression (L/p; an oscillation between psoric anxiety and syphilitic destructiveness). Other examples include: *anger driving to suicide* (L/s) and *anger from homesickness* (*Capsicum*; L/p).

Degrees of Irritability

The **irritable** person (psora) is one who becomes easily peevish for various reasons, even over trifles. Irritability is often accompanied by impatience (choleric temperament). But it is **superficial** and **transient**, not necessarily of short duration (it can last hours, even days) but never intense. He becomes annoyed, impatient, shows it with a sour face, answers in short phrases and then finally, it passes. "Leave me alone" is his attitude. He is always out of humor. You have the impression that you shouldn't bother him, ask questions, or even offer your help (e.g., *Graphites, Causticum*).

But if the patient becomes exasperated, starts shouting, gets red in the face, becomes excited, and manifests his displeasure intensely with pounding his fist on the table, in other words, he explodes, then this is **anger** (sycotic) in the truest sense of the word (e.g., *Nux vomica, Nitric acid, Cuprum, Hepar sulph*).

And when a sudden flare-up of anger gets a tint of the luetic miasm and appears violent, dangerous, and wrathful, this is known as **rage** (e.g., *Tarentula, Stramonium*, even *Sepia*). The rage overwhelms the individual, he loses control and may be driven to kill or commit acts of destruction. The rage also leads to physical destruction: a stroke, a heart attack, malignant hypertension, etc. I read in my local newspaper about a school principal who suffered a heart attack after an altercation with a student. No doubt the principal had syphilitic tendencies! The syphilitic, rage-filled person will throw a chair through the window. If the computer freezes he throws it on the floor, and if his car does not start, he might take a hammer and pound it. When miasmatic states mix with one another, we see rage being expressed in various ways:

- Rage followed by repentance can be categorized as L/p.

- Malicious rage is strictly syphilitic (L).

- Rage coming in paroxysms is mainly syphilitic and secondarily sycotic (L/s).

Degrees of Sadness

Psoric individuals express pure sadness (*Calcarea carbonica*). It can be persistent, but it has a rather peaceful emotional quality, and it drives the person into himself (introspective). Psoric sadness makes us reflect on obstacles to our individuation or self-realization and keeps us in a stagnant condition.

Grief is sycotic because a person externalizes the sadness, even exaggerates it (hysterical) like in *Ignatia*. We do not have to ask, "What is the matter?" because his emotional state will be obvious from his facial expression, his manners, posture, words, etc. The sycotic person's expression of grief is often ostentatious or excessive.

The luetic taint will cause **withdrawal**, hiding, and eventually desire for death (*Aurum*).

Degrees of Disappointment

When a psoric person is disappointed, he will **mull** over his deficiencies, his defects, his meager possibilities. He is immobilized by these things.

The sycotic person, on the other hand, will be driven to **share** his distress with everyone around him. He manifests his disappointment by speaking loquaciously about it, by complaining, by wailing, and by whimpering, in other words, he displays hysterical behavior.

For the syphilitic person, disappointment can be the etiology of a debilitating chronic disease: it may eventually kill the person. I remember an actress who was nominated for an Oscar, and everyone told her she was for sure going to get it. When this did not happen, she collapsed in her bed for a week and suffered afterwards from Chronic Fatigue and Immune Dysfunction Syndrome (*Lycopodium* was her remedy).

Degrees of Joy

Joy is an emotion of pleasure and transcendent satisfaction. For example, I feel joy when I hit a perfect backhand in tennis. In the materia medica, the psoric expression of joy is **cheerfulness**. It is almost an unprovoked reaction, more an attitude of life that a person expresses almost constantly. He maintains a long-term enthusiasm, in an almost corny and childish way. "He is a cheerful person."

cheerful when constipated (*Calcarea carbonica, Psorinum*) and *cheerful in company* are fully psoric expressions.

If cheerfulness is accompanied by dancing, singing, laughing (*Hyoscyamus*), the dominant miasm is sycosis (S/p: mainly sycotic with psoric taint). Another example of S/p is the symptom, *cheerful and foolish*, which can be a characteristic of *Sulphur*. If a patient is, *cheerful when suffering pain* (*Spigelia*), we see psoric cheerfulness combining with the sycosis (S/p), and the person derives pleasure when experiencing pain (morbid pleasure). If we see, *cheerful thinking of death* (*Aurum*), then the dominant miasm is luetic with a psoric taint (L/p).

Mirth is a type of joy characterized by being boisterous, exploding in laughter with ostentatious manners. The person wants everyone to participate in his joy and celebrate the pleasure he feels. They dance, smile, and sing. They may laugh even when they are unhappy or have the symptom: *laughing about serious matters*. In addition, their speech is foolish and hasty, as if intoxicated (*Hyoscyamus*), or the patient plays with words in an intelligent way (*Lachesis*). *Hyoscyamus* displays ostentatious behavior in order to attract attention from others they want to connect with.

Exhilaration represents maximum joy which is almost overwhelming (e.g., *ailments from excessive joy*). The joy completely takes possession of the person, and in this case overwhelms them; they can't control themselves, and as a result, become sick. In states of exhilaration, the cheerfulness becomes an illness, unhinging the person who forgets everything just to rejoice at the event. This may give rise to getting drunk, taking drugs, committing acts of perversion, torturing, abusing others sexually. The exhilarated person develops a sense of omnipotence and a feeling they can do no wrong.

Expressions of Discontent

The symptom of **complaining** describes someone who is always protesting, blaming his unfortunate situation on everyone and everything, giving excuses for his behavior, etc. She is always complaining about the weather (always too hot or too cold), about things that go wrong, about people not behaving as she wishes, about unruly kids, etc. The person seems to be continually irritated and discontent. Typical examples are *Calcarea phosphorica* and *Chamomilla*. They ask for something, you give it to them, and then they throw it away (*capricious*). This is a psoric expression. The psoric person also complains continuously about his health, about trifles, and yet they stay alive for a long time. They are the anxious ones, continuously feeling their pulses, etc. But the complaints are usually only uttered to family and friends (see *Calcarea carbonica* who is a nuisance to those around him).

When the discontent becomes more vocal and extended, we can call it **moaning**: strongly voicing his distress and sadness about things. It is a termed "an audible expression of sorrow, worry, or suffering; grief expressed in words and cries." A typical example is *Kali carbonicum*, one of the most anxious and phobic remedies in the homeopathic materia medica. A person needing *Kali carbonicum* wants tight control over her life but has a hard time achieving it. They frequently harass family members about perceived shortcomings and failures.

The syphilitic manifestation of discontent is the symptom **lamenting**. The person feels anguish about his existence, which seems to be on the verge on destruction. When a syphilitic person laments, they feel as if no good outcome is at all possible. They torment others around them (*Calcarea carbonica* in its syphilitic phase). *Aurum* sees obstructions everywhere and perceives a lack of being validated by others for their efforts (*delusion he is not appreciated*). Even *Nux vomica* laments, but it is all about the other "lazy people" who aren't doing what he says. *Nux vomica* types are in the business of destroying themselves with their indomitable competitive spirit.

As we can see, each symptom has varying degrees of expression that depend on the miasmatic state of the patient. **We must clearly assess why and for what purpose a person expresses a symptom.** We won't have sufficient knowledge about a patient if we just take the symptom *cheerful*, for example. We need to know how the patient expresses their cheerfulness, when and why they feel cheerful, etc. Only in that way will we fully understand all the idiosyncrasies of a patient.

Chapter 16: Additions to Hering's Set of Observations

Failures in Homeopathy

The main reasons for suppression or going against the direction of cure are casual prescribing, the use of too high potencies, too frequent repetition, and prescribing on specifics (*Nux vomica* for constipation; *Cantharis* for bladder infections, etc.) without taking into account the totality of symptoms. The importance of Hering's observations cannot be stressed enough as they will guide the homeopath in his daily practice. In order to really know that the process towards a cure has begun, the homeopath must be able to interpret Hering's observations correctly. Some cases apparently do not follow these observations; see below. In order to know that the process of cure has begun, the homeopath must ask himself two important questions **upon each successive visit** of the patient:

1. Did the natural disease picture return unchanged when the action of the remedy dose ceased?

2. Does the picture follow Hering's observations?

Only when the homeopath can answer "yes" to both questions has the process toward cure begun. At that point, the same remedy, **altered** in potency, should be administered.

Understanding Hering's Observations and Their Pitfalls

First of all, I refer the reader to *Achieving and Maintaining the Simillimum* (p. 192). Based on my clinical observations, I examined Hering's findings in light of modern illnesses and continuous allopathic suppression. By no means did **all my patients' outcomes** follow Hering's observations exactly. That is the reason why they must be called guidelines or observations, **not laws**. Important guidelines nevertheless!

Several ways help us understand and expand on these observations. One way I want to present is the view of Traditional Chinese Medicine (TCM). No definite time-period can be predicted in any case regarding the speed in which these observations will be observed. Every individual heals differently depending on his constitution, his lifestyle, his miasmatic traits, his profession, etc., in other words, depending on Aphorism 5. In a homeopathic practice, the homeopath sees the following basic observations.

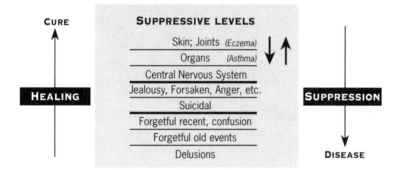

HERING'S SET OF OBSERVATIONS
- Reverse order of appearance of presenting/reversible symptoms
- Healing takes place from more important to less important organs
- Healing takes place from within outwards
- Healing takes place from above to below

As indicated in this diagram, these observations don't all have the same value. The one mostly seen in practice is the **return** of old symptoms. Which symptoms will return? Only the *reversible symptoms*! If the previous or most recently treated layer included destructive, miasmatically syphilitic symptoms, the homeopath cannot expect those symptoms will be able to revert to normalcy. In fact, the more a symptom is related to organic changes and/or destruction, the more slowly it will reappear **if at all** (this again reflects the reactivity of the patient). This also means that symptoms related to gross lifestyle errors (Aphorism 77), except maybe miasmatic cravings, will not disappear: these "pseudo-illnesses" aren't in need of the simillimum but rather of common sense and a change of lifestyle! The symptoms most likely to disappear in the reverse order are especially those that have been suppressed. This is another reason for the homeopath to create a good timeline for the patient, indicating where suppressions have taken place.

When we are talking about reversal of old symptoms or the most recent ones, and how quickly they will be affected by the simillimum, the homeopath must not forget what Hahnemann said:

A 253 In all diseases, especially in quickly arising (acute) ones, of all the signs that indicate that a small beginning of improvement or aggravation that is not visible to everyone, the psychic condition of the patient and his general demeanor are the most certain and revealing. The very beginning of improvement is indicated by a sense of greater ease, composure, mental freedom, higher spirits, and returning naturalness.

> The very beginning of aggravation, on the other hand, is indicated by the opposite —
> a more constrained, helpless, pitiable state with regard to his emotions, mind, general
> demeanor, attitude, posture, and actions, which can easily be seen and pointed out if
> one is attentive but cannot be described in words.

So these mental and emotional changes come **before** the chief complaint disappears and before the reappearance of old symptoms showing further progress toward cure. The homeopath must not forget that dreams, the messenger of the unconscious, might even be the **first** observable change indicating the simillimum. Of course, Hahnemann says the homeopath can only expect these changes **if** the appropriately **small** dose (as small as possible) of the homeopathically indicated remedy has been given:

A 276 ... Excessively large doses of an accurately selected homeopathic medicine, especially if frequently repeated, are, as a rule, very destructive. ...

This aphorism shows again that if you have found the simillimum, you only need to give a very small **dose** (amount) coupled with a high potency (except, of course, in hypersensitive patients and in serious pathology, which require very low potencies).

So even before seeing a disappearance of **any** symptom or the re-appearance of old symptoms, the homeopath should observe Aphorism 253 first.

To put these observations in the right context, here is an example. The homeopath rarely observes symptoms disappearing from above to below in a patient with polyarthritis but rather according to the hierarchy that Hering proposed. If a person has arthritis in the feet and hands, but the feet were affected last, then the feet should improve first, not the hands. The observation, "Last appearing symptoms disappear first" **is predominant over** the observation "from above to below."

After treatment, a dry cough in the lungs becomes a cough in the pit of the throat with mucus production. Although this goes against "from above to below," it is called **exteriorization** of the internal imbalance.

Here is another example of giving the correct interpretation to Hering's observations. The observation, "from above to below," must be taken in its correct context. Indeed, if we have an eczema case all over the body or arthritic symptoms in upper and lower extremities, then indeed disappearance of the complaint from the upper part of body first is the correct direction of cure. Don't forget, however, that the last appearing place where the eczema occurred will be the first to show improvement, **superseding** the above observation.

If we have headaches and heart disease then one might postulate that it is not the correct direction of cure to remove first the headache and then the heart disease since the heart is situated **below** the head. This is taken too literally, however, so here we must follow the rule: healing takes place from more important or Yin organs to less important or Yang organs. This is another example of the hierarchy of observations as shown in the figure above. You can see that this observation is more important than the "above to below" one.

A similar example: the patient originally presents with a case of asthma and mucus in the lung base. After the simillimum (*Kali carbonicum*), he presents with a dry cough and sneezing: this is not called from below (chest) to above (nose) but from interior to exterior (exteriorization). In TCM, the Lungs are a Yin organ and the nose is the door to the Lungs, so the disease gets transferred to the "door" and then will exteriorize and disappear.

The homeopath knows that cure is well underway when there is a reversal of symptoms. This can be a pitfall for the practitioner who may be importuned by the patient. For instance, presume a patient has had constipation for 20 years, regurgitations for 15 years, headaches for 10 years, and asthma for two years. "What is your chief complaint" may be answered "my constipation." (He thinks he has his asthma under control with his allopathic drugs.) Here you risk prescribing based on a disease name and more importantly curing **out of order**! Often, the homeopath observes in the history or timeline that these different disease expressions followed the rule of first attacking the less important organs and then attacking more important or Yin organs, which are more protected from internal and external factors. Here is another reason to treat the most precious, inner organs first before the more superficial ones (Lung versus Large Intestine in this case). Going against this rule leads to palliation where a cure is possible and can therefore transform a curable case into an incurable one. Such interventions are called **suppression**! Boasting about such results is wrong as we find stated clearly in one of Hahnemann's footnotes:

> **A 7** ... A single symptom is no more the whole disease than a single foot a whole man. This method is all the more objectionable because it treats a particular symptom with an opposite remedy (in a merely enantiopathic or palliative way) with the result that it returns much worse than before after a short alleviation.

A homeopath using a superficial or suppressive remedy should be asked to define a real cure and to evaluate whether or not their cases follow Hering's observations.

Additions to Hering's Set of Observations

We can add some other expressions that show the direction of healing. We see healing taking place when symptoms:

• Move from **numbness to tingling and then pain**. This happens in cases of coma and apoplexy. Let me cite an example from Kent's *Lectures on Materia Medica*. He describes a case of an unconscious child who was given *Helleborus*. Under the influence of the remedy, the child comes out of the coma:

> ... you must know what to expect after giving this remedy. The child will become warm and in a few days will return to consciousness—and then what will take place? Just imagine these benumbed fingers and hands and limbs, this benumbed skin every- where. What would be the most natural thing to develop as evidence to the rousing up of this stupid child ... as he comes back to his normal nervous condition, the fin- gers commence to tingle, the nose, ears tingle, and the child begins to scream and toss back and forth and roll about the bed. The neighbors would come and say, 'I would send that doctor away unless he gives something to help that child ... That child is getting well. Leave him alone' (Kent, 1990, p. 517).

Kent is right except he could have done better if he had known about the prescribing techniques of the 5th edition of the *Organon* (published almost 80 years earlier, in 1833!). This child did not need to suffer so. I have treated many stroke patients with the 5th edition method and could ease these patients "back to life" with judicially chosen doses adjusted to the person and his illness, with- out the degree of suffering Dr. Kent describes!

• In cases of musculoskeletal diseases, a cure is established when **diffuse** radiating pain becomes more **intense local** pain, then dull pain, then stiffness and inflexibility, and then freedom from pain. Finally, flexibility and motion return to normal.

• In cases of swollen and painful joints, the pains should be the last symptoms to disappear, and the swelling the first symptom to disappear. The deformities (syphilitic **stigma**) in the joints will never be cured, though the patient will experience better joint mobility and be able to bend them painlessly.

• Moving from multi-organ involvement to a more single organ or system involvement—for example, after the simillimum, a patient with heart trouble and asthma suffers now only from asthma.

• When symptoms move from the center to the periphery.

New Observations

When we speak of the disappearance of the most recent symptoms, disease does not just disappear under the action of our remedy like snow under the sun. Symptoms disappear **only to reappear in a different system, tissue, or organ**. The question is: "Where did they disappear to?" The evolution needs to happen according to **Aphorisms 201 and 202**. Hahnemann tells us in these aphorisms that the internal illness has to go to a place that can be seen and found and at the same time, transferred to an organ that is less precious than the one where the disease came from. In other words, this **transference** of disease, if it follows the direction of cure, has to be to a less important organ (skin and internal skin or mucosa being the most superficial) or else we have suppression, not cure.

You can see from the above that in reality Hahnemann had already formulated some of Hering's observations.

I would like to add some new observations about the direction of cure. Some of them come from TCM, which many times, as a true energetic modality, follows homeopathy's principles and explores the patient's mental and emotional picture as closely as a homeopath. Others come from my study of psychology over the past few years.

• From the front to the back

The Yin and more precious "alarm or Mo or Front Collecting Points" of the meridians are situated on the chest and abdomen. The Yang and Shu or Back Transforming points are found on the patient's back.

I want to add a word about these extremely important points in TCM. The Back Transforming Points and Front Collecting Points are particularly important for the treatment of chronic disease. Indeed, one may go so far as to say that a chronic disease cannot be treated without using these points at some time during the course of treatment. These points become **tender** on pressure and even spontaneously tender when the corresponding organ is diseased.

The Back Shu points transport Qi to the inner organs. Therefore they have a great diagnostic as well as therapeutic meaning and importance. We can also call them **alarm points**, as they warn the patient about discomfort in an organ when they become sensitive. These points affect the organs directly. While I don't expect the homeopath to know these TCM points, working together with a TCM doctor might provide the homeopath with additional information regarding the target organ. The shifting of symptoms from the front to the back of the patient corresponds to the notion, "movement of the symptoms from the more important organs to the less important organs," also expressed in the next observation.

• Moving from Yin to Yang organs

The previous observation refers to the shifting from a more important organ to less important one. So can the homeopath answer to the following questions? Which organ is more important: the large intestine or the small intestine? The gallbladder or the bladder? The kidney or the lung? The stomach or the liver? I have not met one homeopath who could answer these questions, yet the homeopath uses this particular guideline continuously! The homeopath might well learn something from TCM in this case.

First of all, the Yin organs are the most precious organs and have more important physiological functions than the Yang or hollow organs. Therefore, if the clinical patient's picture moves from Yin to Yang organs, the correct direction of cure is assured. The Yin organs are: Liver, Heart, Spleen/Pancreas (one organ in TCM), Lungs, and Kidneys. Note that in TCM, the formation of the brain is a function of the Kidney organ. The Yang organs are Gallbladder, Small Intestine, Stomach, Large Intestine, and Bladder.

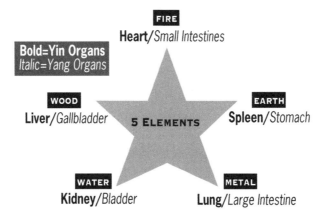

Let's give some examples.

• If the patient's symptoms move from diarrhea (Large Intestine) to dyspnea (Lungs) this is the wrong direction, as the symptoms have gone from a Yang to a Yin organ.

• If symptoms move from bladder polyps to chronic pyelitis: wrong direction! Both are sycotic expressions, so the miasmatic direction cannot help the homeopath but there is a change from a Yang to a Yin organ.

- Cervical spondylitis going to vertigo: wrong direction! Bone and brain affections both belong to Kidney deficiency.

- Recurrent bronchitis (psora) goes now to leucoderma (psora). Good or bad? Good. It is exteriorization, following Aphorisms 201 and 202.

While this first observation is relatively easy to understand, the homeopath finds more difficulty when he must decide between two Yang and two Yin organs affected in the patient. Which of the two is more important? Knowing this will help the homeopath respect Hering's observations while treating such a patient. For instance, a bladder infection disappears and now the patient has an intestinal infection? Good or bad? The solution is found in what the Chinese describe as the **Six Great Meridians**.

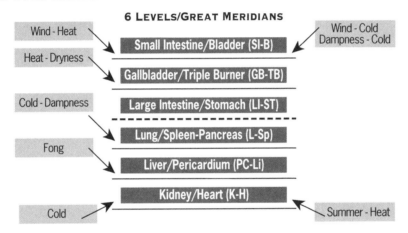

6 LEVELS/GREAT MERIDIANS

In TCM, the meridians are organized in different levels to form a barrier of defense against Exterior Pernicious Qi or telluric or meteorological influences, which, according to Hahnemann's **Aphorism 73** include cold, dampness, etc. Understanding this schema can help the homeopath see whether the direction of cure is correct. Going from the Exterior to the Interior we have the following levels: the SI-B meridian, Tae Yang level, will always be attacked first especially by Wind-Cold and Cold-Dampness causing symptoms such as chills; runny, watery nose; stopped-up nose; no fever, no thirst; sensitivity to cold; stiff neck. Tongue is thin with a white, moist fur.

The next level attacked, if there is an imbalance between the external meteorological factor and the Vital Force (VF) of the patient (either excessive Pernicious Qi or Decreased VF or both) is the GB-TB meridian (Chao Yang) with its main enemy Wind-Heat. Expressions are, most typically, the appearance of **fever**. Also, bitter taste in the mouth; dry throat; stabbing pain in the sides of thorax and chest, and alternating fever and chills. Also, thirst, yellow mucus from nose, and headache. Tongue moderately pink with yellow fur. So the **evolution from a thin tongue, thin white moist fur to swollen tongue with either thick yellow fur or no fur with cracking, redness, and dryness of the tongue as seen on this level, is not in the correct direction of cure!** This is, therefore, another addition to Hering's observations, easy for the homeopath to grasp and observe.

The third level attacked is LI-ST or the Yang-Ming level. The main enemy is Heat-Dryness. Expressions are strong fever, abundant perspiration, strong thirst, and sensitivity to heat. Abdominal distension, belching, gastric pain, foul breath (heat), constipation (heat!), nausea, vomiting, and sinusitis can indicate symptoms of Heat-Dryness. The tongue will appear thick with greasy fur on middle of the tongue.

Note that the first three levels attacked are the **Yang** organs; as we would expect, the Yin or more precious organs are positioned **deeper** and more protected. We see that the SI-B is less important than the GB-TB, which are less important than the LI-ST.

Once we have arrived at the level of the Yin organs, we again will go from less to more precious Yin organs!

The first Yin level is L-Sp (Tae Yin), the enemy is Cold-Dampness. Symptoms are diarrhea, heavy feeling, numbness in the limbs, fatigue, no thirst, no fever, vomiting, sallow complexion, anorexia, bleeding from orifices, uterine prolapse, varicose veins, and hemorrhoids.

A differential diagnosis between the Yang and Yin level is easy:

Yang Ming: fever, thirst, constipation, strong wiry pulse
Tae Yin: no fever, no thirst, diarrhea, slow pulse

The next level is PC-Li, which means Blood Vessels-Liver. This level is especially sensitive to Cold and a mixture of Cold-Heat as well as Fong (Wind), which causes allergies.

Indications of cold attack include: icy cold limbs and fine pulse. A Cold-Heat mixed attack includes symptoms of: dysentery, anal tenesmus, thirst, thoracic oppression, heart pain, and Premature Ventricular Contractions (PVCs). Nausea, vomiting, diarrhea, borborygma, and dysmenorrhea are Liver expressions.

The deepest level, and therefore the **most precious** organs, is K-H (Chao Yin)! The Chinese have a saying: "Any chronic disease will eventually reach the

Kidneys!" One can live with chronic heart failure for a while, but failing kidneys require a speedier intervention with dialysis or transplant. Expressions on this level include: undigested stools, icy limbs, sensitivity to cold, tendency to sleep or insomnia, headaches, memory disturbance, infertility, impotence, diseases of the bones (fragility, caries, slow closing of fontanels), tinnitus, enuresis, palpitations, edema, loss of head hair, lack of will power, and a fearful individual. So if we have a patient who presented with stitching pain in heart and palpitations and now circulatory symptoms arise when exposed to cold (numb fingers, tingling), but stitching pain and palpitations are gone, then we are moving in the right direction.

• From organs to deep meridians to superficial ones (correct direction of cure)

Invasion of superficial channels provokes stiffness and pain along the line of a meridian due to a stagnation of Qi obstructing the channels. If this progresses to the inclusion of organ symptoms (whatever they are according to the organ belonging to the invaded meridian), then we are going in the wrong direction according to Hering. If, on the other hand, symptoms are moving from organ symptoms to the corresponding channel symptoms, a cure is in the works!

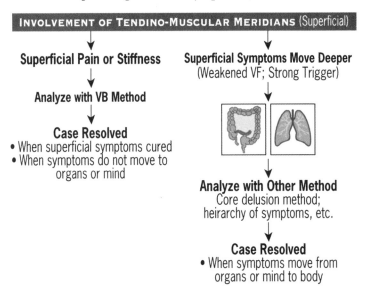

• From empty channel symptoms to full channel symptoms is a sign that the patient is headed toward cure.

CONDITIONS OF CHANNELS	
• **FULLNESS (EXCESS) Qi** Electrical, tearing pain; contractions; cramps; stiffness	• **EMPTINESS OF Qi** Dull, bruised pain; atrophy and weakness of muscles; paralysis and numbess

• **Moving from a syphilitic miasmatic state to a sycotic or psoric one. If cure is immanent, we always see the expressions go from the syphilitic plane (if that's what we started with) to sycosis and then to psoric expressions. This includes the miasmatic nature of dreams!**

The homeopath will find additional guidelines for this observation in the study of the miasmatic expressions (see Chap. 12 and *Hahnemann Revisited*, Section Three).

I want to add the system of miasmatic expressions to Hering's observations. A beginning cystitis (irritation only) is psora, not sycosis. What if the cystitis disappears under our treatment but now the patient shows bladder polyps? This is a sycotic expression and the incorrect direction of cure. Further suppression may lead to cancer (mixed-miasmatic state), again the wrong direction. So it pays to know the diseases belonging to each system and to give them a miasmatic denotation. Going from cystitis to a kidney stone would, for instance, be the wrong direction for two reasons: first, evolution from Bladder (Yang) to Kidney (Yin) and second from psora to sycosis.

Here are more examples from practice. After the simillimum, a teenager went from major anger, rage, and violence to sadness. This is a great improvement and the remedy does not need to be changed. He went from a sycotic state (anger) to a psoric state (sadness).

• From my practice: suppressed gonorrhea when patient was 19 years old. At age 35, bladder polyps were cauterized five times. At age 39, patient developed cancer of bladder (grade IV papillary cancer of bladder) not responding to *tuberculine* (BCG) injections. This case went from an easily curable disease to the sycotic miasm and then to a mixed miasmatic stage (cancer). The patient was cured with homeopathy in one year.

• Evolution from bladder polyps to cataract of the eyes: wrong direction, going from sycosis to the syphilitic miasm.

• Examples from James Compton Burnett (Burnett, reprint 1994, p. 277): A lady with suppressed perspiration, which affected her eyesight; she could only read large print. Suppressing of skin disease leads to angina pectoris. Eczema capitis in an infant was suppressed with local zinc ointment, which caused convulsions from effusion on the brain, and eventually death. Ossified heart from suppressed eczema. Eruption on scalp suppressed, leading to cataracts. Bad skin ulcers "cured" with gold ointment, then ulcers developed on the eyes. These ulcers were cauterized and progression of the disease INTO the eyes led to blindness.

• Example of wrong direction of cure: lady with acne on face for a year. She fell on a bedstead hitting her breast and developed a breast tumor; her skin had never been better!

• Evolution from day sweats to night sweats: loss of precious Yin fluids called by the Chinese, "rob sweat," which robs the body of precious fluids.

• Evolution from bladder prolapse to osteoporosis of the bones: wrong direction, going from under-built sycosis to syphilitic miasm.

• Evolution from stiffness (sycosis) in the spine to tinnitus (psora): good direction.

• Evolution from anemia to vertigo: right direction, from sycosis to psora!

• Someone with bronchitis is remarkably better but now has become obese and lethargic: wrong direction as the patient has gone from psora to sycosis.

• A case of eczema was treated with a homeopathic mixture and *Sulphur* 30C; months later as the eczema disappeared, a painless hard tumor showed up in her breast. Worrisome! From psora to sycosis; also, a painless tumor is often malignant!

• **Moving from a mixed-miasmatic state to a single predominant state (see Chap. 12).**

Cancer and tuberculosis (TB) are always mixed-miasmatic states. Progress from these mixed miasmatic states to a single, predominant miasm is a favorable course. Of course, we also have many cases in which the homeopath sees two different miasmatic expressions but one will be dominant. Evolution towards more expressions of the dominant state will be favorable and obviously easier to treat.

For instance, the patient shows a predominantly psoric state with some syphilitic expressions (P/l): an evolution to pure psora (P) is favorable; a turn to more syphilitic expressions (p/L or L) demonstrates that the disease is being suppressed, not cured.

- **Moving from a mental/emotional attitude to a spiritual attitude or from a spiritual disease ("What is the meaning of my life?") to a mental/emotional one.**

Some aspects of this last guideline might be rather difficult to observe since it requires total honesty from the patient who needs to look into his shadow side and integrate it judiciously into his conscious life. The whole solution will depend on whether the homeopath can find the **motivation** behind the patient's actions and behavior. For instance, someone always "behaves like a gentleman:" always polite, never angry, seeming always understanding and willing to listen. But he does it because he has low self-worth; he is insecure, and he wants to be loved by everyone (longing for approbation). If that same individual acts like a gentleman because he recognizes that it is the right and natural thing to do and not because he wants to be loved by others, then this positive attitude has become part of his nature. In other words, when he has thrown off that mask or persona that hindered his spiritual evolution, he has moved in the right direction and the simillimum has taken effect. He acts like a true individual and is not held prisoner by the question, "What will others think of me?" Jung gives an example in which the patient has dreams of conversing only with higher educated and famous individuals, expressing a secret conscious attitude of haughtiness. Wearing such a mask will stop the person from advancing in his individuation process.

Another similar example is someone who needs *Nux vomica* or *Lycopodium*. They are always helping other people but really doing so because they think, "There might come a moment when I need this man; he might be able to do something for me." They are not true "givers," but only "**exchangers**," or worse, opportunists. They give but they expect to receive in return! If that same individual now behaves as a true philanthropist (and I have known some who literally give the shirt off their back to those in need), then that individual has escaped the enslavement of worldly goods and moved on to higher spiritual spheres. As the homeopath can see, in both examples, we must ask patients the all important question: **"Why and for what purpose are you doing this?"** and hope that we will get an honest answer. If we don't, the patient will betray himself by not achieving cure due to the application of a false simillimum, perceived as such because of defective information, or rather returning to his old behavior more than once as he goes through life since sincerity was not the driving force behind his behavior! Or during case-taking, the patient will contradict himself, giving different answers to the same question, phrased slightly different.

A third and maybe easier-to-detect evolution to the spiritual sphere comes from the emotional plane. More individuals in this century, at around age 40 when they have achieved "everything," suffer from a spiritual disease related to the "meaning of life." The homeopath may see these same people change direction, often with the help of the simillimum, making their own and other people's lives more meaningful. Or the remedy might free the patient from a job that was either self-imposed or encouraged by others for so-called economic/financial reasons. Now instead of being a doctor, he opens a pet store because that's what he always wanted to do. Certainly there will be a great financial adjustment for that person and his family, but here again it is following the right direction of cure. When you start saying, **"What can I do for the world"** instead of "what is the world doing for me," you have progressed one step forwards toward being more complete and individualized; the cure of the disease has started.

• **Moving from a dream with a syphilitic theme to a dream with a sycotic or psoric theme.**

Much more about dream interpretation will be explained in my next book, *Beyond Jung: Dreams, Delusions, and Homeopathy.* Since I have discussed miasms in detail here, I should note that dreams indicate the active miasmatic theme of the patient. A change in the theme of the patient's dreams from a syphilitic theme to a sycotic one is easy to note and can be used by the homeopath as a great indication of direction of cure.

Syphilitic dreams of destruction and self-destruction are very revealing. We must not forget that dreams generally express just the opposite of how patients conduct themselves in their conscious lives, the general rule for dreams. I had a patient, a nun, who was stricken with cancer. True to her Catholic upbringing, she worked to help the poor through organizing support groups and food drives for the homeless. But at night, to her horror, she dreamed of burning the city and killing people. This destructive, hidden, unconscious information was a prelude to her imminent death, which occurred within three months of the diagnosis. The dream revealed the prognosis of her illness. Burning the city may have stood for her own body, predicting her death. It is interesting to mention here that when one dreams of his own death, this seldom refers to actual death. It points rather to a profound archetypal process of transformation in the dreamer.

Psoric dreams involve looking for support and help and carry a more positive prognosis (themes of love, caressing, banquets, singing, gatherings, etc.).

The dreams of **sycotic** patients are dreams of construction (building a house, etc.) but also often relate to their "carpe diem" or seize-the-day attitude. This miasmatic state may be associated with rapidly progressing tumors. Sycotic people often wish to "live it up" and may indulge in risky behaviors like using drugs, casual sexual encounters, even robbery, for the excitement they bring. Sycotic dreams might either reflect this (as in a *Medorrhinum dream of carousing or drinking*) or the opposite, which provides a warning. Other examples would be *Thuja's* dreams of *falling from a height, dying,* or *conscience acquits him of a crime,* or *Medorrhinum's* dreams of *physical exertion from business, death, and disease.*

Dreams can be particularly useful as the homeopath attempts to understand the hidden nature of the syphilitic person and to a lesser degree the sycotic one, as the dreams may reveal facts that would otherwise remain concealed from a practitioner who does not understand the language of dreams and miasms. These miasmatic dreams also provide the homeopath with the certainty of having administered the simillimum to his patient. When he sees the theme of the dreams changing from a syphilitic to a sycotic or psoric theme, he knows he has followed Hering's Set of Observations of Cure.

A Clinical Example

A teenager was taking *Mercurius*; his emotional and physical (colitis ulcerosa) expressions improved greatly as well as his moods and sleep. After some time, he had the following dream: "He was a duck hunter who was randomly shooting at the ducks, but he was greatly bothered by this." In the past he'd had the same dream, but he had enjoyed randomly shooting at the ducks. This sounds like antagonism with his dark side (remorse = psoric), proceeding from a syphilitic state as he gets better.

Furthermore, the homeopath would do well to study *Hahnemann Revisited* (see Chap. 9). The "Pyramid Method" will help one avoid mistakes such as thinking a cure has taken place when the patient's sinuses clear (particular symptom) while he in general has become indifferent to everything, even pleasurable things (an emotional symptom). Such a direction is always wrong, as a particular symptom has less value than a mental/emotional expression.

NEW ADDITIONS TO HERING

- From numbness to tingling to pain
- From diffused to localized pain
- From center to periphery
- From front to the back of the body
- From Yin to Yang organs
- From organs to deep meridians to superficial ones
- From empty channel symptoms to full channel symptoms
- From syphilis to sycosis to psora
- From mixed miasmatic state to single miasm
- From mental/emotional to spiritual state
- From syphilitic dream to sycotic to psoric dream

EPILOGUE

The many-sidedness and variety of homeopathic opinions and approaches in our time is nothing less than astonishing and, at the same time, confusing to student and practitioner alike. When not based on the ground rules set forth by Hahnemann in the *Organon* and *Chronic Diseases*, these approaches amount to confusion and perplexity, rather than granting validity to the various theories. The homeopath must not imitate facets of allopathy. There is, however, **one** aspect in which I would like the homeopath to imitate the allopath: allopaths follow a **uniform** curriculum, misguided though it may be. Homeopaths would do well to first do their best to understand and follow everything that Hahnemann set forth in *Chronic Diseases* and the *Organon*, before embarking on a path of speculation, faith, and pseudo-science. Where, usually, science is not based on the work of one man, but on many individual contributions, homeopathy **is** an exception: Hahnemann completed his science in his lifetime. In my opinion, Hahnemann is one of the greatest scientists who ever lived. He serves as our compass in the patient's life from the cradle to the grave.

The homeopath needs to emphasize **Aphorism 2**, the gentle cure if at all possible, as large doses and high potencies might propel the patient towards a goal he is not ready for. Patients often demand not only fast results, but often "a shock" to their system as a proof that something is happening! We can compare the fragile, often suppressed patient's VF to the butterfly's growth, evolution, and struggle from its cocoon out into the exterior world and eventually on to freedom—when its time has come. Initially the butterfly (our patient) is weak and undeveloped and needs a strong exterior casing (compensations, family support, and the simillimum in the smallest possible dose and highest acceptable potency) for protection. It is still too weak to survive in the world without its shell. When the butterfly (the patient's VF) is strong enough, it will start the journey outward, the process of individuation, freeing oneself from the Core Delusion. If we help the butterfly out by breaking it free from its casing too early (using too high a potency and dose), sooner than it is ready, it will not have the strength to survive, to endure, and to thrive in the outside world. The growth and struggle this butterfly (patient) must endure in a protected environment is part of its evolution and journey and lays the foundation for the butterfly to thrive in freedom. Freedom, if one is not prepared, can be just as imprisoning as prison itself. Homeopathic case management is a true journey of the soul and spirit and takes place on the mental, emotional, spiritual, and physical planes.

Man's quest for individuation is a never-ending process. His Herculean labor must consist of making the unconscious as conscious as possible, integrating his dark side into the light of consciousness. When one deals with the unconscious, one must not be afraid. An unseen foe is the worst: he can assail you from every side. We must understand that our unconscious will always possess the greater store of energy and undigested material, but provides us with something to work on as long as we live. This notion truly corresponds to the never-ending homeopathic treatment, where success is defined as dissolving the Core Delusion, hidden in the unconscious, and integrating it into the whole of the patient's consciousness. This is the definition of the simillimum, as the remedy is based first on finding the Core Delusion, the wellspring from which everything flows!

That most laborious task of becoming an individual, through self-scrutiny and self-fulfillment, is not selfish. It is embracing our own uniqueness and serving as a member of a community. Restraining emotions and guarding secrets are psychological mistakes for which Nature finally visits us with sickness. It is a sin in the eyes of Nature to keep our insufficiency buried in our shadow side and never to confess that we are fallible and human. The first step in freeing oneself from such obsessive complexes is to admit to having them. Then we must follow the Greek dictum, "Give up what you have and then you will receive." This is the motto for the first stage in our homeopathic treatment so that we can detect and dissolve the Core Delusion of the patient! Painful as it may be, what is worthless and inferior belongs to the person as his shadow and gives him substance. How could he cast a shadow if he did not have a substance? I must have a dark side if I am to be whole. In this way, man becomes conscious that he is a human being like any other. And the goal of the liberation of such obsessional chains is not merely intellectual acknowledgment of the facts, but their confirmation by the heart and the actual release of the suppressed emotions with the help of our remedies!

I have written this book hoping to stimulate self-investigation on the part of the homeopath. The homeopath carries a great burden of responsibility to improve himself and his immediate family, and ultimately all those around him who step into the homeopathic process. He has the knowledge for eugenics, but does he apply it?

Often in seminars I ask the question, "Who is taking a remedy?" No more than 20 percent of attendants raise their hand. Why? Is the homeopathic community so healthy? Or are we in denial about our own shortcomings? Or afraid—or worse still, don't we ourselves believe in the awesome powers of the homeopathic remedy? The challenge for the homeopath is to transform himself first, in order to more effectively help his patient—but this is met with scant popular approval. I think the greatest reason is that it is sometimes very painful to make ourselves live up to everything we expect of the patient. It is rather unpopular for the doctor to examine himself. When he does so, he will discover his inferior side, which brings him dangerously near to his patients and perhaps puts his authority in jeopardy. How will he handle a tormenting discovery? But if he does not heal himself, the only solution is for this imperfection to be repressed again. By not resolving his own issues, a doctor can be a harmful factor. I have seen that in my practice. In many cases, his medical diploma is no longer the crucial thing, but his human quality can instead become the decisive factor in the patient's healing.

It is my hope to unify homeopaths under the banner of classical Hahnemannian teachings. Between the realization of this hope and the present, there lies an abyss over which a bridge needs to be built. We should build it stone by stone!

BIBLIOGRAPHY

1. Burnett, J.C. Reprint, 1992. *Best of Burnett.* New Delhi: B. Jain Publishers Pvt. Ltd.

2. Campbell, J. 1976. *The Portable Jung.* USA: Penguin Books Inc.

3. De Schepper, L. 1999. *Hahnemann Revisited: A Textbook of Classical Homeopathy for the Professional.* New Mexico: Full of Life Publishing.

4. De Schepper, L. 2004. *Achieving and Maintaining the Simillimum.* New Mexico: Full of Life Publishing.

5. Frankl, V. 1986. *The Doctor and the Soul.* New York: Vintage Books.

6. Hahnemann, S. 1817. *Materia Medica Pura.* New Delhi: Indian Books and Periodicals Syndicate.

7. Hahnemann, S. Reprint, 1982. *Organon of Medicine.* Sixth Edition. Translated by Jost Künzli, MD, Alain Naudé, and Peter Pendleton. Washington: Cooper Publishing.

8. Hahnemann, S. Reprint, 1997. *Chronic Diseases: Their Peculiar Nature and Their Homeopathic Cure, Volume I.* Translated by L. Tafel, edited by P. Dudley. New Delhi: B. Jain Publishers Pvt. Ltd.

9. Hahnemann, S. Reprint, 2001. *Organon of Medicine.* Fifth and Sixth Editions. Translated by R.E. Dudgeon and W. Boericke. New Delhi: B. Jain Publishers Pvt. Ltd.

10. Hering, C. Reprint, 1992. *Analytical Repertory of Symptoms of the Mind.* New Delhi: B. Jain Publishers Pvt. Ltd.

11. Hering, C. Reprint, 1997. *The Guiding Symptoms of Our Materia Medica.* New Delhi: B. Jain Publishers Pvt. Ltd.

12. Jung, C.G. 1968. *Analytical Psychology: Its Practice and Theory.* The Tavistock Lectures. New York: Vintage Books, A Division of Random House.

13. Jung, C.G. Reprint, 1989. *Collected Works of C.G. Jung, Volume 3: Psychogenesis of Mental Disease.* Bollingen Series XX. Edited and translated by Gerhard Adler. Edited and translated by Sir Herbert Read and R.F.C. Hull. New Jersey: Princeton University Press.

14. Jung, C.G. Reprint, 1991. *Collected Works of C.G. Jung, Volume 9: Archetypes and the Collective Unconscious.* Bollingen Series XX. Edited and translated by Gerhard Adler and R.F.C. Hull. New Jersey: Princeton University Press.

—

15. Kent, J.T. 1911. *Lectures on Homeopathic Materia Medica.* New Delhi: Aggarwal Book Centre.

16. Kent, J.T. Reprint, 1994. *Lesser Writings.* New Delhi: B. Jain Publishers Pvt. Ltd.

17. Maciocia, G. 1989. *The Foundations of Chinese Medicine.* Churchill Livingstone Publishing, London.

18. Roberts, H.A. 1936. *The Principles and Art of Cure by Homeopathy.* New Delhi: B. Jain Publishers Pvt. Ltd., Reprint, 1976.

19. von Boenninghausen, C.M.F. 1908. *Lesser Writings of C.M.F. von Boenninghausen.* A Contribution to the Judgment Concerning Characteristic Value of Symptoms (pp.105-121). Translated by L.H. Tafel and compiled by T.L. Bradford. New Delhi: B. Jain Publishers Pvt. Ltd., Reprint, 1991.

20. Whitmont, E. 1991. *Psyche and Substance.* Berkeley, California: North Atlantic Books.

INDEX

The third companion book to Dr. Luc De Schepper's highly-acclaimed works helps complete the desktop reference trio for the professional homeopath's library:

Advanced Guide for Professional Homeopaths

A companion book to *Hahnemann Revisited* and *Achieving and Maintaining the Simillimum*

Luc De Schepper, MD, PhD, CHom, DIHom, Lic.Ac.

Dr. Luc – homeopath, Hahnemannian scholar, and lecturer – has written the third book in a trio of invaluable desktop reference books for the professional homeopath. Practitioners and students alike know Dr. Luc has devoted years researching the 4th, 5th, and 6th editions of the *Organon*, all editions of *Chronic Diseases*, Hahnemann's *Paris Case Books*, and many lesser known works of von Boenninghausen, Dudgeon, Kent, and other great masters. Dr. Luc continues to share his extensive experience treating the most complex cases in private practice. This new book will help homeopaths overcome the challenging obstacles to their *own* difficult cases using Dr. Lucs' practical guidelines for Advanced Case Taking and Advanced Case Management. Easy-to-read, and very well-organized, the professional homeopath will find themselves referring to its contents quickly and often in the quest for rapid, gentle healing!

Order by Mail

- Full of Life Publishing,
  P.O. Box 31025, Santa Fe, NM 87594

- For INQUIRIES ONLY:
  Phone: 505-982-9273
  Email: **drluc@cybermesa.com**

General Policies

- All orders must be prepaid.
- Check or Money Order accepted.
- Calculate charges for each delivery address.
- Prices and shipping charges may change.
- A $25 fee for returned checks.
- Return within 30 days for future credit only.

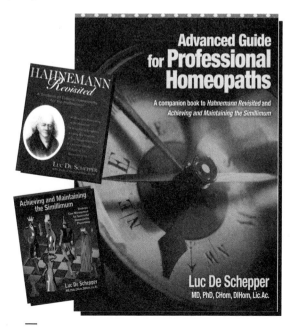

For more information about Dr. Luc's books and the Renaissance Institute of Classical Homeopathy, visit **www.drluc.com**, email drluc@cybermesa.com, or write to:

Full of Life Publishing
P.O. Box 31025
Santa Fe, NM 87594

Shipping in the United States

Shipping and handling: Add $5.50 for delivery in the United States only. For shipping rates outside of the United States, please e-mail Yolanda at **sadiki@cybermesa.com** for a quote. A check must be received before a book can be sent. No exceptions.

> **Make checks payable to:**
> Full of Life Publishing

Order Form:

Advanced Guide for Professional Homeopaths – A companion book to Hahnemann Revisited and Achieving and Maintaining the Similimum

240 pages, hardback $65.00

Shipping: _____

Tax: _____

TOTAL: _____

Shipping Information:

Name: _____

Address: _____

City: _____   State: _____   Zip: _____